# The D.O.'s

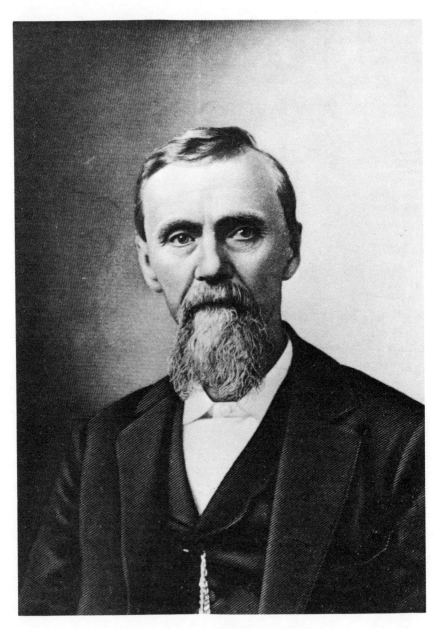

*Dr. Andrew Taylor Still, 1828-1917*

# THE D.O.'s

## OSTEOPATHIC MEDICINE IN AMERICA

*Norman Gevitz*

THE JOHNS HOPKINS UNIVERSITY PRESS
Baltimore and London

Copyright © 1982 by The Johns Hopkins University Press
All rights reserved
Printed in the United States of America

The Johns Hopkins University Press, Baltimore, Maryland 21218
The Johns Hopkins Press Ltd., London

**Library of Congress Cataloging in Publication Data**

Gevitz, Norman.
The D.O.'s.

Includes bibliographical references and index.
1. Osteopathy—United States—History. I. Title.
II. Title: The DO's. [DNLM: 1. Osteopathy—History—
United States. WB 940 G396d]
RZ325.U6G48 1982      615.5'33'0973      82-47978
ISBN 0-8018-2777-9

*For Evelyn Gevitz*

# Contents

# *Preface*

Osteopathic medicine is an enigma within the health care system of the United States. While government estimates suggest that D.O. physicians and surgeons currently serve the needs of upwards of 20 million Americans, little is generally known about the profession. Remarkably, only a few outsiders have attempted to conduct any research on any facet of the movement—this being reflected in the scant mention the subject has received in the social scientific literature.

This book seeks to provide the first comprehensive portrait of the profession, focusing on the impact of ideas and institutions in promoting its early development in the last quarter of the nineteenth century as well as in effecting subsequent changes within its belief system, educational program, and scope of practice. Though written more in a narrative than an analytical style and concerned with a unique rather than a general phenomenon, this work will, I hope, contribute to our understanding of certain key sociological issues as well, particularly the disavowal of social deviance, the problems of status inconsistency and social invisibility, and the consequences of occupational role duplication on professional autonomy.

During the more than six years devoted to this project, several institutions generously extended to me their full cooperation including in most cases the use of their facilities and records: the American Osteopathic Association, Chicago, to whose archives and library I was given ready access; the American Medical Association, also headquartered in Chicago; the American Association of Colleges of Osteopathic Medicine, Bethesda, Maryland; the American Osteopathic Hospital Association, Park Ridge, Illinois; the Chicago College of Osteopathic Medicine; the Missouri State Historical Society, Columbia; the Kirksville (Missouri) College of Osteopathic Medicine; the John Crerar Library, Chicago; the National Library of Medicine, Bethesda; the University of Michigan Libraries; and the libraries of the University of Chicago.

Among the many individuals who aided me in this effort, I especially wish to thank Odin W. Anderson, Ph.D., Professor of Sociology, the University of Chicago and the University of Wisconsin, Madison; Lester S. King, M.D., Professorial Lecturer in Medical History, the University of Chicago; Philip E. Greenman, D.O., Associate Dean and Professor of Biomechanics, Michigan State University College of Osteopathic Medicine; Charles Bidwell, Ph.D., Professor of Sociology and Education, the University of Chicago; and Morris Janowitz, Ph.D., Professor of Sociology, the University of Chicago. I would also like to acknowledge my debt to David Oxman, M.D., who first interested me in the subject, and William Cummings, Ph.D., who convinced me to pursue it as my dissertation topic.

Others I wish to mention for their assistance are: Edward Crowell, D.O.; Anne E. Crowley, Ph.D.; J. Stedman Denslow, D.O.; Mary Jane Denslow; Michael Doody; the late Morris Fishbein, M.D.; Murray Goldstein, D.O., M.P.H.; Leonard Heffel; Elliot Lee Hix, Ph.D.; Robert Kappler, D.O.; Robert Kistner, D.O., M.D.; I. M. Korr, Ph.D.; Norman Larson, D.O.; the late Richard MacBain, D.O.; Nicholas S. Nicholas, D.O.; George Northup, D.O.; Deborah Otis; James Paster; Michael Patterson, Ph.D.; Barbara Peterson; Anders Richter; Linda Stellato; Edward G. Stiles, D.O.; Robert Thompson, Ed.D.; Jackie Wehmueller; and Linda Westerfield.

Finally, I must give special credit to my wife, Melanie Gevitz, for her editorial criticism and emotional strength, and for helping to finance this independent study.

The D.O.'s

# CHAPTER ONE

# *Andrew Taylor Still*

Much of the history relating to the early development of osteopathy has been obscured over time and is the subject of speculation. Like other medical prophets or revolutionaries, the founder of the movement, Andrew Taylor Still, sought recognition as a completely original thinker. In his autobiography, Still maintained that the precepts of his approach came to him in a single moment of inspiration; that no contemporary belief system or practice significantly influenced his theory that most diseases were directly or indirectly caused by vertebral displacements and that elimination of the latter through spinal manipulation would remove symptoms of pathology elsewhere in the body. Although his followers later modified this unlikely interpretation, they did not go far enough in identifying all the intellectual currents that shaped his thought.

Still was born on August 6, 1828, in Jonesville, Virginia, the third of nine children. His father, Abram, had served as a Methodist preacher but at the time of Andrew's birth was supporting his wife, Martha, and their offspring by farming and practicing medicine. However, in 1834, when Andrew was six, Abram once again heard the call, sold his land for the then considerable sum of nine hundred dollars, and moved his family to New Market, Tennessee, where he had received an appointment to preach.[1] In the early decades of the nineteenth century, the Methodist church sent its ministers to follow the steady westward march of the population, making each one responsible for a large geographical area known as a circuit. Often, after spending a few years in one location, a preacher would be transferred so that he might face a new challenge elsewhere.[2] Of these country clerics Horace Bushnell wryly noted that they were "admirably adapted, as regards their mode of action to the new west—a kind of light artillery that God has organized to pursue and overtake the fugitives that flee into the wilderness from his presence. The new settler reaches the ground to be occupied, and by the next week, he is likely to find the circuit crossing by his door and to hear the voice of one crying in the wilderness 'The kingdom of God is come nigh unto you.'"[3]

Andrew's first schooling came in Jonesville at the hands of a man named Vandenburgh. "He looked wise while he was resting from his duties," Andrew recalled, "which were to thrash the boys and girls, big and little, from 7 a.m. to 6 p.m. with a few lessons in spelling, reading, writing, grammar, and arithmetic . . . [pardoning] our many sins with the 'sparing rod.'" At New Market, Andrew attended classes with his older brothers at an academy called Holston College. This institution, much to their relief, was conducted by a man "of high culture, a head full of brains, without any trace of brute in his work." In 1837 Reverend Still was transferred to Macon County in northern Missouri, and for two years Andrew's studies were suspended until his father was able to find a regular tutor. From Macon, the family moved to Schuyler County, and again there was an interruption. But from 1842 through 1848, when he was twenty, it appears Andrew was continuously exposed to formal education.[4]

The family of a circuit rider led an especially rough life on the frontier. There were the periodic moves, and Reverend Still was called away from home on his religious work several times a year for intervals lasting as long as six weeks. The salary provided him by the church was insufficient to provide for his large brood, and Reverend Still had to supplement the preaching income with earnings from his farm and medical practice. As a child Andrew devoted much of his time to chores such as caring for the crops and livestock. He much preferred hunting. On occasion he traveled with his father on ministerial rounds and participated in the camp meetings that the Reverend Still helped lead. At these religious revivals songs were sung, prayers were offered, and conversions were made. The keynote was enthusiasm. In describing this phenomenon, William Sweet observed, "The revival in many instances was accompanied by certain peculiar bodily exercizes, such as jerking, rolling, barking, dancing, and falling. The falling exercize was the most common, and frequently at these great meetings scores, and even hundreds were on the ground, many lying for a considerable length of time either entirely unconscious or semi-conscious. The 'jerks' were also common, though affecting different persons in different ways. Sometimes the head would be affected, twisting it rapidly to the right and left; sometimes it would seize the limbs, sometimes the whole body."[5] In retrospect, it is surprising that these events did not then give Andrew the idea that anatomical displacement was the predisposing cause of most disease.

In 1851 Abram received yet another appointment, this time to the Kansas Territory as missionary to the Shawnee Indians. For the time being Andrew remained behind, married, and began working a farm of his own. Two years and two children later, however, he and his family joined his parents at the Wakarusa Mission. It was here that Andrew decided on medicine as a career and began to study and practice under the tutelage of his father.

When the territory was officially opened up to settlement soon afterwards, the Stills headed for Baldwin, about twenty miles southeast of Lawrence.

This area became the focus of the national debate over slavery. In 1854 Senator Stephen Douglas of Illinois, seeking to open up the frontier to commerce, introduced legislation organizing the land west of Missouri and Iowa as one territorial unit. Southerners opposed the idea because they believed the unit would eventually be admitted as a Free State, thereby altering the existing balance of power in Congress. To win southern support, Douglas amended his bill, calling for the creation of two territories—Kansas and Nebraska—and for the repeal of the Missouri Compromise of 1820, which forbade slavery north of the thirty-sixth parallel. Under his plan citizens of each territory would decide for themselves whether or not they wanted "the peculiar institution." Over considerable northern objection the bill narrowly passed, and President Pierce signed it.[6]

The result was chaos as settlers representing both sides of the issue poured into eastern Kansas. In November, 1854, an election was held to choose a delegate to Congress. Hundreds of proslavery Missourians crossed the border to vote and were successful in selecting one of their own. The next March they returned, establishing a legislature that promptly enacted a slave code. Following this string of setbacks, the abolitionist forces began to rally. Among them was Andrew Still, who became a lieutenant of the movement's leader, James Lane. In 1857 Still was elected to the quasi-legal Free Kansas Legislature, which passed its own set of laws and organized the people to vote down the existing constitution.[7] After three years of continuing political debate as well as intermittent bloodshed, Kansas was finally admitted to the Union as a Free State just prior to the beginning of the Civil War.

At the outbreak of the national conflict Still enlisted in the northern cause and was assigned to the 9th Kansas Cavalry, Company F, as hospital steward, where he was responsible for the procurement of drugs and other medical supplies. In April, 1862, after being released from this service, he returned home, organized his own command, and was commissioned captain. Later Still was transferred to the 21st Kansas Militia with the rank of major. In 1864 he saw action in the successful drive against Confederate forces advancing upon Kansas City.[8] "During the hottest period of the fight," he recalled, "a musketball passed through the lapels of my vest, carrying away a pair of gloves I had stuck in the bosom of it. Another minie-ball passed through the back of my coat, just above the buttons making an entry and exit almost six inches apart. Had the rebels known how close they were to shooting osteopathy, perhaps they would not have been so careless."[9] This battle marked the end of Still's military career. Returning to Baldwin, he resumed his fledgling career as an orthodox physician.

American medicine in the 1850s and 1860s was generally characterized by poorly trained practitioners employing harsh therapies to combat disease entities they understood insufficiently. Before the Civil War the great majority of physicians had never attended a medical school; they either had been trained through the apprenticeship system or were engaging in practice without benefit of any formal background.[10]

The apprenticeship, which could last three or more years, afforded the student a pragmatic education. After reading anatomy and physiology with a preceptor, the trainee would be taught how to diagnose, how to compound and administer drugs, and how to perform common minor surgical procedures. The qualifications of the preceptor were not standardized and, considering the paucity of adequately trained physicians—mainly those who had received their education abroad—instruction was usually poor. Nevertheless, the system itself was quite popular, providing the teacher with a dependable income and a cheap source of labor from the student, who in turn received the knowledge necessary to practice medicine according to public expectations.[11]

After serving an apprenticeship the student could elect to enroll in one of the growing number of medical colleges springing up in the country. The aim of these institutions was to supplement the training already received with formal lectures and demonstrations. Initially, instruction in these schools was brief, consisting of one term of four to six months in length taken in two successive years—and the second term was merely a repetition of the subject matter assigned in the first. The quality of education in such colleges was not good. As they existed to make a profit for their stockholders, their expenditures for equipment, facilities, and instructors were relatively modest.

When A. T. Still began his career in 1854, his medical education consisted of work performed at his father's side and the study of a number of texts in anatomy, physiology, surgery, and *materia medica*.[12] His first patients were the Shawnee. "I soon learned to speak their tongue," he reminisced, "and gave them such drugs as white men used, cured most of the cases I met, and was well received." The Indians also constituted the source of his continuing education in anatomy and pathology, as he made occasional nighttime raids into their burial ground to disinter corpses for dissection. Though his conscience was troubled over this, Still noted that at least his subjects never complained.[13] After studying with his father one of his brothers went on to medical school, but it is not clear whether Andrew did the same.[14] During the Civil War, however, Still received further training in surgery, learning the latest procedures for amputating a limb, removing a bullet, and cleansing and dressing a wound. Andrew later maintained that his duties far exceeded those subsumed under his title of hospital steward.[15]

Medical thought and practice in these years was highly speculative and largely empirical. Most American physicians believed that disease was due to organic decomposition, climate, heredity, and mechanical injuries. The germ theory, which had lost favor in the first half of the century, was just beginning to be revived. More than cause, the practitioner was preoccupied with effects. Many physicians thought of disease as the sum total of symptoms and reasoned that the faster each was removed (the temperature lowered, pulse restored to normal, bowels evacuated, or stomach purged), the more rapid the patient's recovery would be. Those disorders bearing common attributes tended to be treated by similar or identical methods, serving only to encourage the use of panaceas such as bloodletting.

Playing an instrumental role in this trend was Benjamin Rush (1745-1818), a signer of the Declaration of Independence and perhaps the most influential American physician of his time. Rush believed the basis of all disease was physiologic tension, particularly of the veins and arteries. In his treatment of this condition, he found the drawing of blood most effective. In fact, bleeding the patient for any acute illness became his practice and teaching, and in later years he even claimed that often the only equipment the physician needed for house calls was the lancet.[16] The results of moderate bloodletting were dramatic and seemed palliative: a sudden drop in temperature, profuse sweating, and a sense of calm. Some practitioners believed that utmost benefits were achieved when patients were bled to unconsciousness. Although the theory upon which Rush based his practice was discredited shortly after his death, yellow fever, cholera, typhoid, typhus, smallpox, croup, and enteritis were popularly treated by bloodletting, which was conscientiously performed by the majority of orthodox physicians in America until about 1870.[17]

Another widely employed panacea was calomel, a mercury compound that acted as a powerful cathartic. So popular was this remedy in the mid-nineteenth century that it was commonly referred to as "the Samson of the *materia medica.*"[18] Since most physicians felt that in treating internal ailments a cleansing of the system was desirable, calomel was often prescribed and not infrequently administered in conjunction with bloodletting. In large doses it was responsible for some dangerous side effects. As Risse has noted:

> Within a few days after ingestion, severe stomatitis with excessive salivation appeared. Patients had ulcerated lips, cheeks, and tongue, soreness and inflammation of the gums, plus loosening and frequent loss of teeth. Some unfortunate children died with perforation of their cheeks, bucal gangrene, and osteomyelitis of the maxillary bones. Generally there was gastric pain associated with vomiting and gastrointestinal cramps after ingestion of the

calomel. In some cases bloody diarrhea occurred which was ascribed to the disease. . . . The larger doses were considered to have a so-called sedative effect, no doubt because of the more severe systemic consequences of the mercurial poisoning.[19]

Because the drug would not readily pass from body tissues, several years of even intermittent use would produce a cumulative reaction.

In addition to calomel other toxic pharmaceuticals of dubious value, such as arsenic, antimony, tartar emetic, lobelia, strychnine, and belladonna, were generally employed. A small number of truly useful agents were available in this area: quinine for malaria; colchicine for gout; opium for pain; and digitalis for dropsy. But as Ackerknecht notes, each was utilized in the treatment of a host of other ailments, where their introduction was either of no assistance or even harmful.[20]

Such symptomatic management was not accepted by all orthodox physicians, however. As early as 1835 Jacob Bigelow introduced the concept of the "self-limiting disease," which he defined as "one which received limits from its own nature and not from foreign influences; one which after it has obtained [a] foothold in the system, cannot in the present state of our knowledge be eradicated or abridged by art."[21] Through a careful study of the drastic, or what was commonly called "heroic" measures then in use, Bigelow demonstrated that none significantly improved the patient's chances for recovery. Though the article that announced his beliefs received favorable notices in the medical press, the reaction of most of Bigelow's contemporaries was indifference. Heroic therapy continued unabated.

In 1860 Oliver Wendell Holmes, Sr., M.D., declared in frustration, "If the whole *materia medica* as now used could be sunk to the bottom of the sea, it would be all the better for mankind—and all the worse for the fishes."[22] Holmes subsequently became the object of severe criticism, as did others who attacked the prevailing practices. In 1863, when William Hammond, the surgeon general of the United States, issued an order removing both calomel and tartar emetic from the Union Army supply table, the doctors revolted. Hammond was blasted by the medical societies and his decision was never enforced.[23] Though physicians could appreciate the arguments in favor of the self-limiting disease, it was not practical for them to follow the logic of this approach by excluding their powerful remedies. Many felt it was their role to act; their patients' expectations were other than to have them sit by passively, simply watching and waiting.

In the early Kansas years the heroic approach to medicine combined with the unavailability of effective remedies helped produce a short life expectancy. Malaria was probably the leading cause of adult mortality. Though the benefits of quinine were widely known to the first generation of settlers, the drug was quite expensive and often difficult to secure. Also decimating the population was smallpox. Many Kansans doubted the efficacy of vaccination, which had been popularized by Edward Jenner (1749-1823), and never bothered to submit themselves to the simple procedure. Some feared that vaccination was dangerous and would only spread the disease. Other scourges for which there were no effective therapies—typhoid fever, pneumonia, scarlet fever, typhus, dysentery, and meningitis—were all frequent visitors to the pioneers' homes.[24]

In treating clients suffering from these and other conditions, Still employed such generally accepted drugs as castor oil, gamboge, aloes, calomel, lobelia, quinine, and soap pills. Though he may have, as he said, harbored some doubts about their relative value at the beginning of his practice, this did not stop him from prescribing them.[25] Only when tragedy struck his own household in the spring of 1864 did Still begin seriously to question the practice of regular medicine. "War," he wrote, "had left my family unharmed; but when the dark wings of spinal meningitis hovered over the land, it seemed to select my loved ones for its prey." Following the interdiction against treating one's own close relatives, Still summoned nearby physicians, who took immediate charge. He recalled the scene:

> Day and night they nursed and cared for my sick and administered their most trustworthy remedies, but all to no purpose. The loved ones sank lower and lower. . . . God knows I believe they did what they thought was for the best. They never neglected their patients and they dosed and added to and changed doses, hoping to hit upon that which would defeat the enemy; but it was of no avail. It was when I stood gazing upon three members of my family . . . all dead from the disease spinal meningitis that I propounded to myself the serious questions "In sickness had God left man in a world of guessing? Guess what is the matter? What to give and guess the result?"[26]

While Still would not abandon orthodox medicine per se for another ten years, this personal loss inspired him to evaluate various alternative systems of practice which had already arisen. "Like Columbus," he said, "I trimmed my sail and launched my craft as an explorer."[27]

### Alternative Medical Systems

The first significant challenge to orthodox medicine in America was led by Samuel Thomson (1769-1843), a crude, self-educated individual who postulated that all disease was due to the body's inability to maintain its natural heat. As therapy he rejected bloodletting and calomel, employing instead six botanical remedies that caused the patient to sweat and vomit. Thomson attacked the legitimacy and integrity of the medical profession on several grounds, arguing that the motive of the regulars was often to obtain a larger fee by prolonging illness; that formal education was an unnecessary prerequisite to practice; and that licensing laws passed on the grounds of protecting the public against "quacks" were only the means by which one group could monopolize the healing arts. Though they were ridiculed by the regulars, Thomson's attacks appealed to many Americans in the age of Jackson, when the virtues of the common man were extolled and special privilege accorded anyone was frowned upon.[28]

Thomson, however, was not loathe to obtain his own special privilege, securing a patent on his system of medicine and selling family rights for its use at twenty dollars apiece under a slogan stating that every man could be his own doctor. Mobilized by Thomson into "friendly societies," his followers lobbied intensively in state legislatures against existing licensing laws that restricted medical practice to the regulars. By the 1840s almost all of these statutes were repealed, amended, or otherwise made ineffective. This meant that for the next several decades anyone could practice medicine practically anywhere in the country without fear of being prosecuted.[29]

A distinctly different and more intellectual threat to the medical establishment was presented by homeopathy, which was adopted by thousands of educated physicians in the United States who had been trained in the orthodox tradition. This movement was originally launched in Germany by Samuel Hahnemann (1755-1843), an erudite university graduate who, like Thomson, opposed the standard remedies then in use. In the 1790s Hahnemann began performing experiments on himself, recording the physiological reactions produced by various drugs. The first drug he tested was cinchona bark from which quinine is derived. He found that if he ingested it while perfectly healthy, his body would manifest several of the symptoms of malaria. This led him to conclude that the drug best able to cure a given disease was the one that produced most of its symptoms in a well person. Other agents were tested by Hahnemann and his followers, who found the use of such homeopathic or "like cures like" remedies most effective, especially when administered in extremely small amounts.

The homeopaths developed their own comprehensive *materia medica* and offered their system as a substitute for the practices of orthodox doctors, whom they labeled *allopaths*. The allopath, declared Hahnemann, was one who would offer treatments that produce completely opposite effects of the disease when administered in health. In subsequent decades, however, the term *allopath* lost its original signification and became a convenient label used by all alternative medical movements in describing "regular" or "orthodox" physicians.

The rapid growth of homeopathy can be easily understood. Its followers did not administer toxic levels of the standard pharmaceuticals of the day;

nor did they employ bloodletting. Thus patients had only to bear the disease, not the treatment as well.[30] Even Holmes, its arch critic, would note that homeopathy "has taught us a lesson of the healing faculty of nature which was needed, and for which many of us have made proper acknowledgements."[31]

Before 1860 most American homeopaths were educated in regular medical colleges and learned the Hahnemannian system upon graduation. After the Civil War, as a result of being expelled from membership in orthodox societies and institutions, they built their own schools and hospitals and formed their own associations. The instruction in these colleges was as complete as that in allopathic schools of the day, the two differing only in the content of their *materia medica* and approach to patient care. With respect to facilities, staff, and clinical opportunities, most homeopathic institutions were, according to Rothstein, equivalent to their orthodox counterparts.[32]

Due partly to the increasing popularity of homeopathy, a schism occurred within the Thomsonian ranks. Where the founder wanted to restrict his followers' therapeutic armamentarium to the six drugs he used and opposed any formal medical training, several of his more sophisticated supporters could not agree. They wished to experiment with all available botanicals as well as any other agent that held promise. Under the leadership of Wooster Beach (1794-1868), this group broke away and opened their own colleges, eventually adopting the name *eclecticism* to describe their desire to shun all restrictive tenets or principles. In actual practice, however, the eclectics who rejected most drugs of mineral origin and substituted resinous medicinals for the regulars' alkaloid pharmaceuticals did so purely on dogmatic grounds. As for the schools they established before and after the Civil War, these were academically poor, and most of the physicians they produced were not as well trained as those graduating from their competitors' colleges.[33]

Whatever their respective strengths or shortcomings, unorthodox practitioners flourished as the century progressed. At their apex, they collectively represented approximately 15 percent of the entire physician population; the homeopaths were located principally in the cities and the eclectics mostly in rural areas.[34] It is difficult to establish how much influence these systems had on regular physicians, who soon abandoned their heroic measures, but certainly their success in attracting a sizable number of patients gave pause to many in the orthodox ranks.

In studying these reform movements, Still came to the realization that they generally offered a less harmful regimen to their patients than did the regulars. This was not good enough; they were, to his way of thinking, just as empirical. "First I tried the ability of drugs as taught and administered by allopathy," he once observed, "then noticed closely the effect from the schools of eclecticism and homeopathy. I concluded all was a conglomerate mess of conjectures and experiments on the ignorant sick man from the crown to the heel. I learned that a king was just as ignorant of the nature of disease as was his coachman, and the coachman no wiser than his dog."[35] The central issue in medicine, he would maintain, was not which drug to use and in what dosage, but whether drugging itself was a scientific form of therapy.

No less important was his moral concern. As a Methodist, Still adhered to the temperance teachings of his church, which was but one of several groups that supported the prohibition of alcoholic beverages during the middle decades of the nineteenth century.[36] After the war he asked himself, if drinking was sinful, should drugs be classified any differently? "I was not long in discovering," he reflected, "that we had habits, customs, and traditions no better than slavery in its worst days and far more tyrannical." For this he laid the blame on the physician, proclaiming the cause to be ignorance of "our schools of medicine." He observed, "I found that he who gave the first persuasive dose was also an example of the same habit of dosing and drinking himself, and was a staggering form of humanity wound hopelessly tight in the serpent's coil."[37] Thus increasingly convinced that internal medication of any kind was immoral as well as invalid, Still would continue his explorations in a different direction.

### Drugless Substitutes

This was an era in which a number of drugless systems had appeared and gained some degree of success in drawing adherents. An early entry was the "popular health movement" led by Sylvester Graham (1794-1851), a temperance speaker who in the 1830s began to lecture against gluttony, improper dress, sexual permissiveness, and medicines while arguing in favor of bathing, fresh air, exercise, and diet. Graham maintained that man was heading toward physical degeneration by not living according to the dictates of Nature's laws. Some of his arguments appeared most reasonable. Bathing in this period was not regularly practiced, the common diet was unbalanced, and clothing for women was unnecessarily restraining. Although the farmer was constantly exposed to sunlight, fresh air, and exercise, the commercial and leisure classes were not; indeed, many believed such a life to be unwholesome or demeaning. On the other hand, much of Graham's advice, notably his ramblings on the supposed evils of too frequent sexual encounters, was based upon what his biographer, Shryock, has called a "sublimated puritanism."[38]

In 1839 he published a collection of lectures which became a best seller.

Graham claimed that following the principles outlined in his book would make drugs and physicians unnecessary because first, his supporters would be less likely to get sick; second, if they did fall ill, they would not be as severely affected; and third, by allowing their bodies' natural self-restorative powers to operate, they would recover more quickly.[39] Graham ruled out certain "unhealthy" foods: meats, fresh milk, eggs, coffee, tea, and pastries. His substitutes were invariably bland and tasteless; the most well known of these was a cracker that still bears his name, originally designed to curb not only one's hunger but also one's sexual appetite. Graham's critics were quick to point out that his ultimate goal seemed to be to take enjoyment not only out of the kitchen, but out of the bedroom as well.

Though Graham argued that his system was all inclusive, a number of his followers as well as others soon began to frequent the offices of another group of drugless practitioners, the hydropaths. An Austrian peasant by the name of Victor Priessnitz had discovered that cold water seemed quite effective in treating many of the chronic ills of both man and beast, most notably gout and rheumatism. Within a short time his approach caused a small sensation in Europe, and several sanitaria were opened on the Continent for the teaching and practice of his methods.

Hydropathy was exported to America in the 1840s. Two medical schools were established, and by the mid-1850s at least twenty-seven spas were in business, mostly in rural areas of the East and Midwest, where the water was believed to be the most pure. The cure primarily consisted of drinking the precious fluid as well as enveloping one's body in it. According to Legan, "A sheet of cotton or linen dipped in cold water was spread on several thick woolen blankets. . . . Over the whole was thrown a feather bed, and the patient remained in his cocoon from twenty-five minutes to several hours, depending upon the seriousness of his condition and his ability to work up a good perspiration. Next the victim was unswathed and cold water was poured over him, or he was immersed in a cold bath and finally briskly rubbed dry."[40] Quite clearly, "heroic" therapy could be practiced by drugless healers as well.

Still's familiarity with Graham's notions and hydropathy can be traced to his early manhood, when a utopian colony following a combination of these ideas was established near the Shawnee Mission.[41] This experiment did not last long, but while it existed the Reverend Still had to be called on several occasions to care for those not responding to or suffering from the regimen. Undoubtedly Andrew was not especially impressed then or later with these methods. Yet Still came to believe that the drugless approach was the right one. It was only a matter of seeking out a system that could provide a more logical basis for reliable diagnosis and efficacious treatment. Towards this end, Still would find considerable guidance in the principles and practice of magnetic healing.

In 1774 Franz Mesmer (1734-1815), an Austrian physician, postulated that an invisible universal magnetic fluid flowed throughout the body and that too much or not enough in either a part or the whole was one major cause of disease, particularly nervous disorders. The only rational course of treatment, therefore, was to restore the fluid to its proper balance. This could be accomplished by making passes over the body with magnets or his hands. Mesmer was not the first to heal through the use of touching; rather he was the first to fashion this approach into a coherent system of medical practice.[42]

Many of his early cures through this method were greatly publicized, and soon he was attracting patients all across Austria. His success there, though, was short-lived, as pressure from the medical community of his native Vienna forced his departure for the more enlightened Paris. In the French capital, Mesmer's practices became more irregular. Instead of seeing clients separately and discreetly, he formed groups and ministered to several patients at once. Often he employed a huge indoor tub with extended "magnetized" rods. Those gathered would bathe together, placing the afflicted parts of their bodies against the metal protrusions, until Mesmer materialized. While an orchestra played solemn music, he entered the room dressed in a flowing, lilac-colored robe and touched his patients as he passed. This was designed to bring each individual to a near seizure-like state, which, according to Mesmer, was often necessary to achieve catharsis. The tub was not his only healing site. Clients would also be treated outdoors, under "magnetized" trees or beside "magnetized" rocks.[43]

As Mesmer's practice gained popularity, two special commissions were created in 1784 to investigate the relative merits of his claims. One of these groups was appointed by the French Academy of Sciences and included in its ranks Benjamin Franklin, Jean Sylvan Bailly, and Antoine Lavoisier. This committee declared that a "magnetic fluid" did not exist and that Mesmer's cures were only the result of suggestion, and intimated that the morals of women undergoing such treatment were being threatened. In an induced seizure, they argued, females could become easy targets for se-duction.[44] With the appearance of this study, Mesmer's personal influence waned. Some of his followers, however, who still believed his basic prin-ciples to be valid, abandoned the tub and other questionable procedures and tried to gain respectability. In succeeding decades, they made progress. In 1831 a somewhat favorable report on the subject was issued by the French Adademy of Medicine, and backhanded support came later, from James Braid's (1795-1860) writings on what was eventually called hypnosis.[45]

Magnetic healing was brought to the United States in 1836 by Charles

Poyen (?-1844), who gave a series of public lectures in Boston and took on a number of students, training them in massage and other methods then thought to be useful in restoring fluid balance.[46] Poyen's activities helped stimulate considerable interest in the subject, and though his stay in America was relatively brief, the seed he planted was soon able to sprout without him.[47] One of those who allegedly heard Poyen lecture was Phineas Parkhurst Quimby (1802-65), who afterwards established a practice consisting largely of verbal suggestions combined with light stroking of the body. Though Quimby's writings were not published until long after his death, he was an influential figure during his lifetime, serving as physician, teacher, and inspiration to Mary Baker Eddy (1821-1910), the founder of Christian Science, and as the intellectual fountainhead for the loose confederation of religious groups known as "New Thought."[48]

The most well known magnetic healer prior to the Civil War, however, was Andrew Jackson Davis (1826-1910), who was also the leading American exponent of spiritualism.[49] In the first volume of his massive tome, *The Great Harmonia* (1850), Davis sought to combine both belief systems. Conceiving of the body as a machine, he maintained that health was simply the harmonious interaction of all man's parts in carrying out their respective functions. This was due to the free and unobstructed flow of "spirit." Any diminution or imbalance of this "fluid" would cause disease.

Like others before him, Davis placed emphasis on healing with his hands. Of particular interest is his management of asthma, which consisted in part of vigorous rubbing along the spinal column.[50] While this type of treatment constituted but a small feature of Davis's practice, later magnetic healers, perhaps influenced by the attention given the spine by such orthodox physicians as Bell, Magendie, and Hall, made extensive use of it. One of these was Warren Felt Evans (1817-89), whose name is most often associated with "Mind Cure."[51] In his book entitled *Mental Medicine* (1872), which went through fifteen editions, Evans noted, "By the friction of the hand along the spinal column, an invigorating, life-giving influence is imparted to all the organs within the cavity of the trunk. The hand of kindness, of purity, of sympathy, applied here by friction combined with gentle pressure, is a singularly effective remedy for the morbid condition of the internal organs. It is a medicine that is always pleasant to take."

These sentiments were echoed in the book *Vital Magnetism* (1874), written by another popular healer, Edwin Dwight Babbitt (1828-1905). He specifically mentioned convulsions, apoplexy, sunstroke, headache, muscular complaints, common rheumatism, and paralysis as disorders capable of cure through spinal treatments. It is not known whether Still read these works by Davis, Evans, and Babbitt; however, he was well aware of their message. A letter cosigned by him to the *Banner of Light* indicates that he was a reader of the spiritualist- and magnetic-healing-oriented journal that published articles and advertisements by each of these practitioners within its pages.[52]

Though Still never embraced all of the ideas of these contemporaries, a number of the central tenets of magnetic healing made a strong impression on him: the metaphor of man as a divinely ordained machine; health as the harmonious interaction of all the body's parts and the unobstructed flow of fluid; and, of course, the use of spinal manipulation. His most significant departure from them would be over the nature of the fluid. While for the remainder of his life he spoke obliquely of the physiological role of magnetic energy, it was free flow of blood, he believed, that constituted the key to health.[53] "I proclaimed," he later wrote, "that a disturbed artery marked the beginning to an hour and a minute when disease began to sow its seeds of destruction in the human body. That in no case could this be done without a broken or suspended current of arterial blood, which by nature was intended to supply and nourish every nerve, ligament, muscle, skin, bone, and the artery itself. He who wished to successfully solve the problem of disease or deformity of any kind in every case without exception would find one or more obstructions in some artery or vein."[54]

In June of 1874, Still severed his ties to regular medicine, an action that shocked his community. Many of his friends and relatives, in response to his "laying on of hands," questioned his sanity, while the local minister, seeing him as an agent of the devil, had him "read out" of the Methodist church. Still asked for permission to explain his practice at nearby Baker University, a school that he had helped build, but the privilege was denied.

Effectively ostracized in Baldwin, Still traveled to Macon, Missouri, to visit a brother and see if public acceptance of his newly adopted methods would be any better. It was not. After staying there a few months, treating but a small number of patients, he moved on to Kirksville, situated in northeast Missouri, where to his surprise "three or four thinking people" actually welcomed him.[55] The city then had a population of eighteen hundred and was the commercial capital of Adair County, which had a total of some thirteen thousand inhabitants. In a local paper, the *North Missouri Register,* he advertised himself: "A. T. STILL, MAGNETIC HEALER, Rooms in Reid's building, South Side Square, over Chinn's store. Office hours—Wednesday's, Thursday's, Friday's, and Saturday's from 9 am to 5 pm with an intermission of one hour from 12 pm to 1 pm."[56] Though his practice in this new locale was not particularly successful at first, he was comforted by the fact that there was no organized harrassment by either the clergy or the local physicians. Still was also able to go about his business without serious interference from the state. The law governing the medical arts in Missouri was weak, and prosecutions few.[57] As a result of the tolerance he had initially been shown, he moved his family there the following May.

In the fall of 1876 Still contracted typhoid, the effects of which left him an invalid for more than six months. After he fully recovered, Still realized that his local clientele would be too small to support his loved ones as well as pay off the debts incurred during his illness. In desperation he applied for an army pension but was turned down due to technicalities.[58] As it was necessary to expand his population base, Still decided to become an itinerant like his father before him, practicing in several communities throughout the state for extended periods, while his wife and children remained in Kirksville. For the next few years Still's earnings barely kept pace with his expenses. On various occasions his relatives offered to help him out financially if he would return to orthodox medicine, but Still adamantly refused.[59]

### The Lightning Bonesetter

Sometime during the late 1870s Still became interested in bonesetting, another form of manipulative practice limited to the field of orthopedics. In deciding to learn these techniques, he may have hoped to be able to treat a wider range of disorders, thus giving him the potential of substantially increasing his patient load and his income.

Bonesetters were an ancient if not respectable group of healers. In England they had enjoyed a relatively unfettered practice among the common people who could not afford a regular physician and who often had difficulty locating one willing to take their case. However, bonesetters could also count on the patronage of members of the upper classes, including royalty, who believed that their particular talent, passed down from one family member to another, was a gift that transcended formal book learning.[60]

In addition to reducing dislocations, bonesetters also manipulated painful and diseased joints, thinking they too were caused by a "bone out of place." Physicians ridiculed their crude diagnoses and dismissed their claim that such treatment was of any value. Nevertheless, some patients with restricted joint mobility that remained unrelieved by trained orthopedists were apparently benefited upon receiving manipulative therapy administered by such "quacks." Some physicians assumed that these clients were only hysterics, or that the patient and the bonesetter were in collusion to embarrass the doctor in charge; but in 1867 Sir James Paget, himself a most distinguished surgeon, startled his colleagues by announcing that he believed there were joint maladies that bonesetters, regardless of their inaccurate diagnoses, were able to cure and that only through a searching investigation of their techniques could the relative value of such treatment be fully understood. "Few of you," he admonished his educated brethren, "are likely to practice without having a bonesetter for a rival and if he can cure a case which you have failed to cure, his fortune may be made and yours marred."[61]

In 1871 Dr. Wharton Hood, an acquaintance of Paget, published a book in England and the United States based upon his experiences as a bonesetter's apprentice. As he described it, the bonesetter's technique constituted "the art of overcoming by sudden flexion or extension, any impediments to the free motion of joints that may be left behind after the subsidence of the early symptoms of disease or injury." The conditions for which Hood believed this type of treatment useful were: cases of stiffness, pain, and adhesion following fractures and sprains of one or more of the bones forming a joint; rheumatic or gouty joints; displaced cartilages; subluxations of the bones of the carpus and tarsus; displaced tendons; hysterical joints; and ganglionic swellings.[62] However, he cautioned that bonesetting was only successful where the ability of joints to rotate had not already been permanently destroyed.

While most of their activity was limited to manipulating the extremities, bonesetters, as Hood noted, were being resorted to by people who were "complaining of a 'crick' or pain, or weakness in the back, usually consequent upon some injury or undue exertion, and . . . these applicants are cured by movements of flexion and extension, coupled with pressure upon any painful spot." Often during these maneuvers a "popping" or "clicking" sound would be emitted by the spinal joints, which many times convinced the patient that a cure of the problem had been effected.[63]

Bonesetters could be found in America since the colonial era—the most priminent practitioners were the Sweet family, who held forth in the New England area for nearly two hundred years.[64] How widespread such manipulators were elsewhere in the country can only be guessed at. One physician in 1884 estimated that in every city in the United States "may be found individuals claiming mysterious and magical powers of curing disease, setting bones, and relieving pain by the immediate application of their hands."[65]

It is not clear how Still learned to become the "lightning bonesetter" he would advertise himself to be throughout the 1880s. Though he could have come across Hood's book, it seems more likely that his knowledge was derived from observing the work of another practitioner in the field.[66] However he learned these methods, Still soon afterwards made an important discovery, namely, that the sudden flexion and extension procedures peculiar to this art were not limited to orthopedic problems, and that they constituted a more reliable means of healing than simply rubbing the spine.

About 1880, he would later recall, "An Irish lady . . . had asthma in bad form, though she had only come to be treated for the pain in her shoulder. I found she had a section of upper vertebrae out of line, and I stopped the pain by adjusting the spine and a few ribs. In about a month, she came back to see me without any pain or trace of asthma. . . . This was my first case of asthma treated in the new way and it started me on a new train of thought.[67] Soon he was handling headache, heart disease, facial and arm paralysis, lumbago, sciatica, rheumatism, varicose veins, and an increasing variety of other chronic ailments, all by manipulating vertebrae back into their "proper position." In accounting for his success, Still would synthesize some of the major components of magnetic healing and bonesetting into one unified doctrine. The effects of disease, as the former said, were due to the obstruction or imbalance of the fluids, but this in turn was caused by misplaced bones, particularly of the spinal column. At this point, Still had given birth to his own distinctive system.

In the next decade Still traveled across Missouri touting his new approach. According to one eyewitness:

Sometimes he would leave Kirksville with barely enough money to pay carfare and go to some town with a bundle of probably a thousand bills, get them scattered, after which he would give an exhibition of setting hips, probably on a public square, in a spring wagon or ox-cart. Of course, he would be looked upon as some mysterious being, crazy, or at least daffy; but with his intuitive insight, he would pick out a cripple, or someone with a severe headache or some disease that he could cure quickly, and demonstrate before the anxious crowds.[68]

Often, Still had a difficult time getting his ideas across. He saturated his speeches with an odd collection of metaphors, parables, and allegories which left many listeners bewildered.[69] His unusual attire—a rumpled suit, a slouch hat, his pants tucked inelegantly in his boots—caused some to look rather than listen. Many times he could be seen on the streets clenching a long wooden staff he used as a walking stick while toting a sackful of bones over his shoulder. Not surprisingly, such behavior led people to form one of two opinions: either he was an eccentric genius or a deranged old man. Nevertheless, as one follower noted, "the impression left was usually a good one."

One or more of his sons would often travel with him and assist in treatment. Harry Still later observed:

I believe I would be safe in saying that in the six months we practiced in Hannibal [1884-1885] we accumulated a dray load of plaster paris casts, crutches, and all classes of surgical appliances. We went from Hannibal to Nevada, Missouri where the state insane asylum is located. Here we made fully a hundred cures. . . . I remember one interesting case. The lady had been in the asylum for several years. It seemed she had lost her mind suddenly while playing a piano. Father examined her neck and found a lesion of the atlas. In less time than I have taken in the telling, the girl was as rational as ever. Strange to say, the first thing she said was "Where is my piano and music?" She was anxious to finish the piece she had started playing three years before."[70]

Unusual recoveries such as this one gradually spread the "lightning bonesetter's" reputation. By the late 1880s his scheduled trips to various towns caused considerable local excitement. In Eldorado Springs he had to reserve sixteen rooms to treat the crowds that had gathered. People reportedly came to Nevada City from upwards of 150 miles away, complete with tents in anticipation of a long wait.[71] Still was now becoming a charismatic figure.

Paradoxically, it was only after he had obtained notoriety elsewhere that the people of Kirksville began to patronize him in large numbers. One incident in particular helped change his image. The young daughter of the town's Presbyterian minister, J. K. Mitchell, had for some unreported reason lost her ability to walk. After her child had been treated without apparent benefit by other local physicians, Mrs. Mitchell, in desperation, asked her husband to allow Still to make an examination. The reverend adamantly refused. Nevertheless, while her husband was away on an extended trip, the child's mother called for Still, who proceeded to adjust the girl's spine. When Mitchell returned home his daughter walked down the stairs to greet him. With the good pastor now singing praises to Still's name, the social barriers that had long prevented "the lightning bonesetter" from treating "decent folk" were lowered.[72]

As a result of his new-found respectability, Still decided to make Kirksville his permanent home. In 1889 he established an infirmary there to carry on his work. Soon patients from great distances were seeking him out. "It was a problem," said one follower, "how best to take care of the people that were flocking to him. . . . Many of those who came were pronounced hopeless by other physicians. Some of them were hopeless. But he was able to cure enough . . . to keep adding to his reputation and his fame which extended into ever widening circles."[73]

All of this success would convince Still that he had discovered a new science of healing. What he lacked was only a proper designation for it. "I began to think over names such as allopathy, hydropathy [and] homeopathy," he recalled. Eventually this led him to "start out with the word *os* (bone) and the word pathology, and press them into one word—osteopathy."[74]

# CHAPTER TWO

# *The Missouri Mecca*

Having named his new system of medicine, Still decided it was time to share his discovery with others. In 1892 he opened the American School of Osteopathy, charging his students five hundred dollars for several months of personal instruction. Upon completion of the specified course, students were to be awarded a certificate stating they were diplomates in osteopathy, or D.O.'s.

A few months before classes were to begin, Still had the good fortune to meet Dr. William Smith (1862-1912), a thirty-year-old Scottish physician who was in town on a business trip. Smith had been trained at Edinburgh and had studied for several additional years on the Continent; his background was in stark contrast to that of the self-taught country doctor.[1] After hearing of the "d---d quack" from a local regular, he decided to investigate osteopathy on his own. "I sat entranced," Smith wrote a few years later of his first encounter with Still. "The theories he introduced were so novel, so contrary to all I had read or heard that I failed to follow his reasoning. Arguments as to their impossibility were simply met with the one statement: 'But it is so; there are no "ifs" and "ands" about it, I do what I tell you and the people get well.'"[2] After visiting several boarding houses around town and seeing the results that had been obtained under such care, Smith became convinced that something of value was being imparted. As he wanted to learn more, Smith accepted Still's offer to teach him everything he knew; in return, the young doctor would serve as an instructor in Still's proposed school.

On October 3, 1892, classes began with fifteen men and three women in attendance. The ages of the pupils ranged from eighteen to sixty-five. Some held college degrees, others had nothing more than a common school education. All of them, however, had been direct or indirect beneficiaries of Still's ministrations. Each morning for four months Smith drilled the group in anatomy without the benefit of a cadaver to demonstrate upon. This problem was compensated for in part by his lecturing, which, according to one of his students, "was of such an impressionable type that one who listened to him could virtually look into the human body with

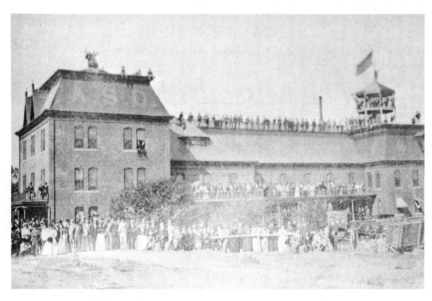

*The American School of Osteopathy (1898)*

his mind's eye and see all its numerous functions."[3] Smith's role was also symbolic. As one early student shrewdly noted, "'Bill' furnished the 'front.' He 'looked good' to the people and inspired confidence in infant osteopathy."[4]

Following their daily anatomy lesson, students spent the afternoons in the infirmary with the "old doctor," as he was affectionately called. Still thought of himself as a natural philosopher who taught principles, not an academician who recited dry facts. Students had to pick up what knowledge they could by listening to his extended metaphors and his sometimes rambling commentary. One of his followers declared, "He rose to the lofty heights of his conceptions of life, health, disease and medicine by the purest of intuition. He wiped the slate of knowledge, as it were of much if not most of the accepted, accredited teachings of the day, not only in the field of medicine, but also in science, religion, ethics, politics, and endeavored to begin his thinking upon any and every subject with the new data of pure forms, built out of his imagination, with little regard or discomfort if his excursions took him sheer in the face of every accepted belief and profession."[5]

"The human body," Still told his students, "is a machine run by the unseen force called life, and that it may be run harmoniously it is necessary that there be liberty of blood, nerves, and arteries from their generating point to their destination."[6] He illustrated the significance of this basic principle with a colorful analogy:

Suppose in far distant California there is a colony of people depending upon your coming in person with a load of produce to keep them from starving. You load your car with everything necessary to sustain life and start off in the right direction. So far so good. But in case you are side-tracked somewhere, and so long delayed in reaching the desired point that your stock of provision is spoiled. If complete starvation is not the result, your friends will be at least poorly nourished. So if the supply channels of the body be obstructed, and the life-giving currents do not reach their destination full freighted with health corpuscles, then disease sets in.

Given such circumstances the osteopath would "remove the obstruction by the application of the unerring laws of his science, and the ability of the artery for doing the necessary work will follow. As a horse needs strength instead of a spur to enable him to carry a heavy load, so a man needs freedom in all parts of his machinery with the power that comes from the perfection in his body, in order to accomplish the highest work of which he is capable."[7]

The highlight of the students' day was watching him operate. According to one, "We would hold the patients in position while Dr. Still . . . worked upon them, explaining to us as he treated why he gave this movement in one place, and a different moment in another. He would tell us what it would mean to the nerves from that particular region if muscles were 'tied up' or a bone was out of line." In diagnosing these conditions, a student explained, Still taught "that we should place the patient on his side and then pass our hands carefully over the spinal column from the base of the spine, noting temperature changes as we went along. Should there be a lesion along the spine, where nerves may be disturbed, it would easily be detected through an abnormal coldness or hotness of the tissues at that point."[8]

Often students could observe the progress of patients over an extended period of time, as the afflicted usually agreed to remain in Kirksville for a minimum of one month. "Remember," Still told them,

that when many of you come to me you are not the most choice kind of patients. Remember the company you have kept before coming here. You have been with doctors who blister you, puke you, physic your toenails loose, fill your sides and limbs with truck from hypodermic syringes. You come to me with eyes big from belladonna, backs and limbs stiff from plaster casts—you come with bodies suffering with all the diseases the flesh is heir to. Remember you have been treated and dismissed as incurable by all kinds of doctors before coming to us, and if we help you at all—we do more than others have done.[9]

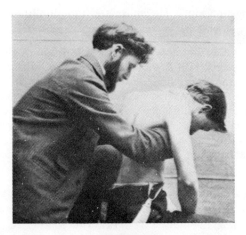

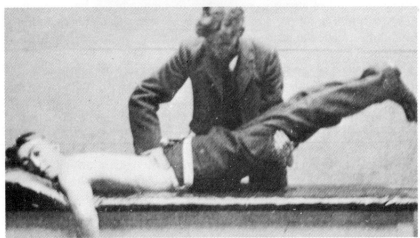

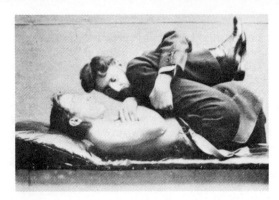

*Dr. Dain Tasker demonstrating manipulative techniques (1903)*

While in Kirksville each supplicant had to obey the interdiction against the use of liquor. "We do not wish to treat habitual whiskey tubs," Still declared. "This rule must be strictly obeyed by all patients, and those who feel that they cannot conform to it had better stay away." Internal medications were taboo as well: "No system of allopathy, with its fatal drugs should e'er be permitted to enter our doors. No homeopathic practice with its sugar coated pills, must be allowed to stain or pollute our spotless name. . . . Osteopathy asks not the aid of anything else. It can 'paddle its own canoe' and perform its works within itself when understood. All it asks is a thorough knowledge of the unerring laws that govern its practice and the rest is yours." Still left no doubt that he considered alcohol and other drugs a moral evil. Indeed, often his crusade centered more on them than on the benefits of manipulation: "Was God ever drunk? Was Nature ever intoxicated?" He once estimated that 90 percent of his work involved overcoming the effect of such poisons upon the body.[10] If one had faith in the wisdom and completeness of God's design, Still maintained, one had to see that the use of drugs was not just immoral, it was unnecessary as well.

### The Word Spreads

Throughout Missouri and elsewhere, more people were beginning to learn of Still's activites from sensationalized newspaper accounts. The *St. Louis Democrat* called Kirksville "the great Mecca for invalids, particularly those suffering from bone disease, dislocations, and similar afflictions. To and fro there surges a throng of ailing humanity sincere in purpose as the Eastern devotee who kneels at the tomb of Mohammed. But the results accomplished are not visionary or fanciful, they are real and practical. Marvelous even unto the miraculous are some of the cures and yet they are all treated in a natural and scientific manner." The *Des Moines Daily News* noted in its columns that Still was "performing remarkable cures in a very simple way," while the *Nebraska Daily Call* declared that osteopathy had deservedly "won a substantial claim to the confidence of all classes of invalids." Some reporters told their readers that they arrived in Kirksville hardened skeptics and left true believers. One Iowa journalist confessed, "It was an experience for the correspondent which removed from his mind every vestige of incredulity to the truth of these innumerable testimonials favorable to osteopathy and the eminent doctor." The editor of the *Bethany* (Illinois) *Echo* even submitted himself for treatment and later told his readers, "If you have an ailment which our doctors cannot successfully treat we advise you to go to Kirksville and be cured."[11]

All of these and other favorable stories were subsequently reprinted in a monthly tabloid Still published called the *Journal of Osteopathy,* which was mailed to friends and relatives of patients in Kirksville as well as to local papers throughout the Midwest. Average issue circulation rose from several hundred in 1894 to more than eighteen thousand two years later.[12] With this publicity greatly increasing the number of patients, more trains had to be scheduled through town to accommodate the traffic. Special reduced-rate fares were soon established by the railroads for those who required shuttle service. New hotels were built and boarding houses flourished. Storekeepers were pleased to find that their shops were constantly crowded. Seemingly everyone in town was prospering from Still's work.

Still's representatives met each train that pulled into the station, greeting clients, arranging accommodations, and setting up appointments with his staff. One reporter noted of the infirmary:

> Everything is managed as smooth as clockwork. . . . The almost constant ringing of electric bells announcing that room so and so is ready for another patient, the great discipline with which patients take their positions near the doors of the operating rooms when their turn is "next," the incessant click of the typewriter as it wades through the immense correspondence, the frequent "helloing" at the telephone, and the general counting room appearance of the business office, impress the visitor that besides an understanding of the human mechanism and laws of health, a thoroughly organized business system is required to do the great amount of work accomplished daily by this wonderful institution. There are now over five hundred patients and when it is remembered that treatment is given each patient from one to three times a week, it is not difficult to understand that the ten operators are kept moving.[13]

Of those who came to the infirmary, one journalist observed:

> Almost every phase of society, nearly every section of the country, and certainly quite, if not all the ills to which human flesh is heir, were represented. There was the laboring man, the business man, and the professional man; there was the working girl, and the society favorite; there was the anxious husband with the invalid wife, the loving mother with her cripple child; there were scores on crutches and in invalid chairs; there were others who were compelled to depend on strong arms and tender hands. One thing they possessed in common, and that was a beaming countenance that indicated confidence, an expectancy, if not already a realization of a bettered condition.[14]

Contemporary accounts indicate that the majority of incoming patients were suffering from chronic, noninfectious disorders. In a sample of forty-nine patients cited in one issue of the *Journal of Osteopathy,* ten were diagnosed as having some form of joint dysfunction, seven a nervous disorder, six asthma, five partial or complete loss of a special sense, three bowel difficulties, and the remainder had other long-term health problems.[15] One enterprising patient took a survey of 109 fellow sufferers. Of these, 61 percent reported having some form of "spinal complaint"; the second most common problem was bone or joint maladies of the extremities. A different point of view was provided by a reporter from Godey's Magazine, who wrote, "From my own observation I think that a majority of the patients were afflicted with nervous troubles and paralysis."[16]

Many clients were willing to discuss their cases openly and give testimonials to the newspapers. F. H. Barker was a Methodist minister from Kansas who had fallen from a train, severely wrenching his neck; he subsequently developed sore eyes and ultimately became blind. Barker claimed to have seen oculists in three states before coming to Kirksville. After undergoing treatment at the infirmary for five weeks he reported that he had no more pain and that his eyesight was almost normal. R. W. Neeley of Franklin, Kentucky, developed a serious case of "heart disease with nervous prostration." "When I landed in Kirksville," he told the press, "I could not walk across the room without holding to chairs. I felt like toppling over at every step. From the very first treatment I began improving, and can't express it better than to say I feel like a young colt in a clover field on a bright spring morning." Mrs. J. T. Christian, the wife of a Baptist preacher, brought her seven-year-old son, who had suffered for three years from what had been diagnosed by two physicians as hip joint disease. According to the newspaper account, "As soon as he was placed on the operating room table here a partial dislocation of the hip and spine were discovered. They were at once reduced without weights, braces, plaster of Paris, or any other paraphernalia; and now the boy is able to go anywhere on crutches, without his brace, feels no pain, the abscesses having disappeared, and will soon be well again." After being treated for several weeks for a chronic case of sciatica, J. W. Blocker of Dark County, Ohio, was only bothered by an occasional pain in his ankle. A Mr. English from Quincy, Illinois, was deprived of the full use of his right leg and arm and other parts of the body by what was diagnosed as a "spinal affection." After treatment he was walking about without crutch or cane. Asked by a reporter if he believed in miracles, Mr. English replied, "Not often, but I am a firm believer in osteopathy."[17] Perhaps the most publicized early case was that of the son of United States Senator Foraker who was sent to Kirksville with what had already been diagnosed as "valvular disease of the heart." As his physicians had given up any hope for the child's survival, there seemed little to lose by trying Still, and indeed, under his care, the symptoms of the condition gradually disappeared. Because of the national attention given the Foraker child, several among the political and economic elite came to Kirksville and further spread osteopathy's good name.[18]

The events taking place in Kirksville did not escape the attention of the state medical association, which determined to put a stop to them. The association's first action appears to have been taken as early as 1889, when it pushed through the legislature an amendment to the existing healing arts law which read, "Any person who shall by writing or printing or any other method publically professes to cure or treat diseases, injuries, or deformities by manipulation or other expedient, shall pay to the state a license of $100 a month." This, however, was unenforced.[19] Later in 1893, after Still secured his school charter and began teaching his first class, the regulars, in cooperation with the homeopathic and eclectic societies, introduced a bill into the House rendering it necessary for those practicing osteopathy to be graduates of a reputable medical school. Apprised in time of this move, Still's students and patients began a petition drive that was active throughout the state. Hundreds of protesting letters and telegrams poured into the lawmakers' offices, leading to the defeat of the bill by a wide margin.[20]

After winning this battle Still and his followers went on the offensive, seeking specific legislation that would guarantee the legal right of D.O.'s to practice within Missouri's borders. One of Still's legal advisors, P. F. Greenwood, linked osteopathy to the aspirations of midwestern populism. In reference to the three established schools of medicine, Greenwood drew a religious analogy: "Suppose Baptists, Methodists, and Cumberland Presbyterians were the only recognized churches to save souls in this state and we were assured the legislature intended to rid the people of the Commonwealth from the doctrines and teachings of heretics? Would you call that class legislation? A monopoly of free gospel certainly. Then is not our medical class legislation as bad? I hold that if medicine is a science that no legislation is necessary to uphold or protect it." Greenwood continued his defense of osteopathy by stating that he trusted people to "have sense enough to employ whatever school or class of medical practitioner they wish. That we have the testimony of intelligent gentlemen and ladies, sufficient to satisfy anyone if they can be satisfied by human testimony that pain and suffering, diseases and dislocations have been successfully treated by the school of osteopathy, that it is a science, and all it asks is an equal chance in the race of life. If it is not a science the challenge is open to the world to disprove it. It asks but one favor and that is the modification and change of the unfair medical laws of this state."[21]

Leading the medical opposition was a prominent orthopedic specialist from St. Louis by the improbably coincidental name of A. J. Steele. He argued that every cult, regardless of its methods, professes cures. Osteopathy was simply no different from Christian Science, magnetic healing, and the waters of Lourdes. As to osteopathic theory, it was entirely invalid. Steele pointedly asked,

> Is the honest, scientific work of educated men and acute observers of the past ages down to the present to be thus ruthlessly set aside? Do our studied research in pathology and therapeutics go for naught? Strange is it not that of the thousands of skeletons carefully examined that frequent examples of misplaced bones have not been discovered, if such truly is the cause of all disease? We see patients daily recovering from sickness and disease in whom no effort has been made to reduce misplaced bones, showing that the *causus morbi* did not lie in that direction. *Per contra*, we have had cases where dislocation and deformity did exist, for example of the spine, and neither organic nor special disease followed—the soft parts accommodating themselves to the displaced bones and the normal functions being well performed.[22]

Some osteopathic followers responded by challenging their critic's competence, claiming that a number of his unsuccessfully treated patients came to Kirksville only to return home free of their affliction.[23] William Smith, however, admitted that there was due cause for the skepticism of his fellow M.D.'s:

> If a man, a physician, comes to Kirksville and hears what he will hear and tries to reason it out on the basis of what he learned in medical school, there is only one conclusion to which he can come: that osteopathy is a fraud and a delusion, a gigantic humbug which is taking from the pockets of the sick and afflicted thousands of dollars monthly. BUT, if the enquirer will just approach the matter as though he knew nothing (and after four years experience of osteopathy let me tell any doctor that he knows very little), take nothing for granted, accept no statement for or against osteopathy; but just interview a dozen patients and accept them as reasonable men and women and not as hysterical persons, half-fitted for the lunatic asylum, nor utter and gratuitous liars, he is BOUND as an honest man to come to the conclusion as I did that there are still some things in the healing art which are not known to the medical profession. Let him examine further and he will find results obtained quite impossible under treatment with medicine. Then let him inquire of the patients who tell him in their stories, how many doctors had declared their recovery impossible, and then, and not until then, let him make up his mind as to whether or not osteopathy is a fraud, its practitioners humbugs and its supporters liars. If all these persons claiming to be benefited are liars where can the profit come in from running the business? To pay such an army of liars would consume the capital of a state. If they are hysterical why did not their doctors cure them?[24]

Despite vigorous medical opposition, the legislature ultimately voted in favor of the osteopathy bill. This measure called for D.O. graduates to present their diplomas for registration to their county clerk, who in turn would issue a certificate making them eligible to treat disease through the hands. The osteopath would not be required to pass any test or attend classes for any set length of time.

All of this went for naught. When the proposed law reached the desk of Governor Stone he decided to veto it on the grounds that osteopathic practitioners were insufficiently educated. "Medicine is a science," he declared. "A judicious practice of it requires a good general and fundamental education, and a thorough knowledge of all the departments of medicine: anatomy, physiology, chemistry, pathology, therapeutics, practice, etc."[25] In other words, if osteopathy wanted equal treatment under the law, it had to conform to the academic scope adhered to by other practitioners of the healing art.

Stone was excoriated by the bill's advocates, but the substance of his objections went unanswered. Indeed, there was little Still or his followers could say in justifying what then constituted osteopathic education and standards. From 1892 through 1896, three classes had been graduated. The length of training varied from nine to eighteen months and consisted of lectures in anatomy, osteopathic principles, and technique. Still believed other subjects were unnecessary. Once, he stormed into a class, raced to the blackboard, and wrote on it in large letters NO PHYSIOLOGY and then left the room. Anatomy, in his view, was the sole medical certainty. There was no need to bother with the theories and speculations of other branches of medicine.[26] The American School of Osteopathy's first charter and early board meetings show that Still wanted to include surgery as well as obstetrics as part of the curriculum, but at that time these subjects had not been introduced.[27]

Stone's veto and the urgings of Smith and others who had previously argued that the D.O.'s training was incomplete finally convinced Still that he had to make changes. By the end of 1896 he had formally lengthened the course of study to four terms of five months each, and at dedication ceremonies of a new college building he announced, "I am now prepared to teach anatomy, physiology, surgery, theory and practice, also midwifery in that form that has proven itself to be an honor to the profession."[28] Several months later he published a more detailed course outline that also included histology, chemistry, urinalysis, toxicology, pathology, and symptomatology.[29] Thereafter Still's supporters maintained that every subject covered in a standard medical college, with the exception of *materia medica,* was taught at the American School.

After Still had thus complied with the governor's major objections, his followers revised their bill and resubmitted it to the legislature, which speedily passed it. On this occasion, the D.O.'s did not face an executive veto. In the interim Stone had left office, and his successor, Lon Stephens, signed the measure into law on March 3, 1897.[30] When word reached

Kirksville, pandemonium reigned while the entire population set aside a day for celebration. "The morning was ushered in," according to one newspaper account, "by the firing of anvils in honor of Governor Stephens, the legislature, Dr. Still and everybody connected with the fight. Bells rang and whistles blew. Anything that would make a big noise went. Residences, stores, shops were decorated, the big osteopathy building was covered with flags and bunting inside and out, and the whole city donned its best fourth of July attire."[31] As students marched down the streets they cheered:

> Rah! Rah! Rah!
> Missouri passed the bill
> for A. T. Still
> Goodbye Pill
> We are the people
> of Kirksville.[32]

### The New Faculty

The passage of this law brought more matriculants, now confident that their time and money would not be wasted. Indeed, within a few years there were seven hundred full-time students in attendance.[33] This growth, coupled with the expansion in the curriculum, forced Still in 1897 and 1898 to engage additional teachers. Among those he found to assist Smith and himself were C. W. Proctor (1859-1949), holder of a Ph.D. in chemistry; Charles Hazzard (1871-1938), a university graduate who also held a D.O.; Carl P. McConnell (1874-1939), who after earning his osteopathic diploma received an M.D. at a homeopathic school; and the three Littlejohn brothers: J. Martin (1865-1947), who had a law and divinity degree from the University of Glasgow and a Ph.D. in political science from Columbia; James (1869-1947), who held both an M.D. and a Ch.M. from Glasgow; and David (1876-1955), who earned a Ph.B. at Amity College and his medical diploma from a Michigan medical school. All had benefited personally from osteopathy or had a close relative or friend who had been helped.

Although this group remained intact for a comparatively brief period, its effect upon the development and course of the movement was significant. Where Still had built his system largely upon the principles and practices of magnetic healing and bonesetting, his new faculty relied upon more reputable sources of knowledge.[34] Joint manipulation, after all, had a lengthy orthodox tradition, and others before Still had postulated that disturbances or displacements of vertebrae could cause symptoms elsewhere in the body.

In ancient Greece frictions—a form of massage—were employed to treat a wide range of ailments. Some of the Hippocratic writings deal extensively with the subject, one work noting that "the physician must understand many things and frictions not the least of all . . . for frictions can bind a joint that is too loose, and loosen a joint that is too rigid." In later centuries manipulation was practiced by Roman healers, but with the Empire's decline, the art disappeared from Europe. When it was finally rediscovered in the Renaissance, it took a relatively minor position in therapy compared to drugging. However, over the course of the next several centuries it would be promoted by a host of distinguished physicians including Gerald von Swieten (1710-72), who advocated manipulation as a general measure to increase blood circulation. "The vital powers," he said in words that foreshadowed Still's, "may be increased by friction to any extent without any foreign addition to the body."[35]

Throughout the 1800s a small group of English and American doctors who employed massage in their practice tried to alert the medical profession to the modality's value through a number of books and articles. Balfour (1819), for example, recommended it in rheumatism and sprains; Bacot (1822) considered it helpful in treating several surgical diseases; and Cleobury (1825) manipulated in cases of contracted joints and lameness from various causes. Later in the century, S. Weir Mitchell (1872), as a result of his Civil War hospital experience, relied on manipulation to treat many traumatic nerve and muscle injuries, and by 1877 he included neurasthenia, hysteria, and locomotor ataxia among its indications.[36] William Murrell (1886) added constipation, poisoning, lumbago, and sciatica to the list; G. L. Pardington (1886), migraine; and A. J. Eccles (1887), constipation.[37] The most extensive clinical research on the subject was carried out by Douglas Graham (1884), who, citing the results of fourteen hundred of his own cases as well as those handled by others, reported success in uterine disorders, hemiplegia, infantile paralysis, writer's cramp, muscular rheumatism, sprains and joint afflictions, rheumatoid arthritis, glaucoma, and in catarrhal affections of the nose, pharynx, and larynx.[38]

Some advocates of massage worked on spinal complaints. George H. Taylor (1884) noted:

> It has been pretty clearly proved that the circulation of the blood, and therefore the proper nutrition of the spinal bones, are quite dependent on the flexibility of the spine, which displaces and replaces the vertebral nutritive fluids, much as the functional use of muscles secures their nutritive support. It follows that the proper therapeutics in vertebral disease is not suspension of the flexibility of the vertebrae by mechanical restraint. . . . It has been practically demonstrated that exactly the opposite course is therapeutically indicated and that the most successful treatment of vertebral disease consists essentially in judicious use of this physical property of elasticity and flexibility.[39]

While their practices paralleled Still's, neither Taylor nor other proponents of massage gave the spine any central theoretical role in disease; nor did they focus upon it in directing their overall therapy.

Their success in treating a number of disorders went virtually unchallenged by their fellow physicians, but massage failed to be integrated alongside *materia medica* in the standard medical school curricula. Most American and English M.D.'s simply felt it was beneath them to administer treatment with their hands, let alone enter a field dominated by unorthodox healers. This attitude did not necessarily apply to other countries. "French, German, and Scandinavian physicians," Douglas Graham acidly remarked, "often apply massage themselves without any thought of compromising their dignity."[40]

The popularity of manipulation in these nations was largely the result of the efforts of Peter Henry Ling (1776-1839), a fencing master who combined body mechanics and gymnastics into what was popularly called "Swedish Movements." Ling's procedures were designed for both prophylactic and therapeutic purposes. His exercises were divided into active and passive types, the former accomplished by the patient alone or with equipment, and the latter requiring the assistance of a trained specialist who would manipulate the patient through flexion and extension procedures. Though first dismissed as being of no value by the Swedish medical community, Ling's approach was later observed to secure satisfactory results in cases where medication had been found wanting. As a consequence, a fair number of Northern European physicians learned his techniques and began applying them in chronic, and even in some acute, cases. One bibliographic study of the literature reveals that hundreds of articles and many books on this system were published during the last half of the nineteenth century.[41]

In examining the massage and Swedish Movements literature, Still's new faculty recognized the similarity of the systems to osteopathy in the type of diseases successfully treated and in some of the techniques employed. However, they firmly believed that their own approach was more specific in terms of diagnosis and therapy. "Upon the whole," Charles Hazzard remarked,

> these manual systems compare with osteopathy as does the shot gun with the rifle. They produce excellent results by the "shot gun method" of general manipulation, while osteopathy works with the definite aim of finding the obstruction to health and removing it. It is unavoidable that, if such a comparatively "hit and miss" method of massage can secure excellent results as a curative means, osteopathy, with its definiteness, must generally far exceed massage in results. It also follows that osteopathy must generally work more quickly and easily than massage in such cases as the latter could reach, and that it must succeed in a large class of cases beyond the power of these

manual systems, since to this class belong so many disease conditions depending upon some removable obstruction not noticed by them.[42]

While emphasizing the supposed shortcomings of massage and Swedish Movements, Still's faculty was not loathe to borrow a number of their underlying principles, particularly the importance of treating muscles and working manually to restore physiologic harmony in the absence of palpable anatomic displacement. In addition, advocates of these two systems provided them with experimental evidence on how manipulation cures. Zubludowski, for example, found that massage increased electrical contractility of the muscles; Hopadze showed how it sped assimilation of food; Golz proved that it aided the circulation of the blood; J. K. Mitchell reported that it could produce an increase in red blood cells; and von Mosengeil found that manipulation promoted lymphatic absorption.[43]

The one area in which Swedish Movements and massage research could not materially assist the faculty was in explaining why Still and his followers were obtaining their results by focusing predominantly on the spine. They found a partial answer in neurophysiology. In 1828 a Scottish physician, Thomas Brown, wrote an article in which he argued that pain about an internal organ could be caused by a disturbed vertebra that shared a common nerve supply. He called this phenomenon "spinal irritation."[44] In succeeding years his theory gained currency and a number of books dealing with the subject were published.[45] One who accepted a similar principle but who did not use the term *spinal irritation* was the English surgeon and anatomist John Hilton (1804-78). In his popular and influential treatise *Rest and Pain,* first published in 1863, Hilton spoke instead of "sympathies," which covered the relationship between visceral pain without accompanying inflammation and "sore spots" about segmentally related vertebrae. To treat this type of pain, said Hilton, one must only treat the spine, which he did with rest and restriction of mobility.[46] While Still's staff seemed only vaguely aware of the doctrine of spinal irritation, they were quite familiar with Hilton's work and often cited his case studies in their lectures.[47]

Charles Hazzard and J. Martin Littlejohn argued by analogy that if referred pain could be produced by displaced vertebrae other remote symptoms, as Still argued, could be caused by them as well. Many of the nerves originating from the spine are connected to the sympathetic ganglia, whose function is to regulate blood flow to the various organs. Furthermore, many contemporary scientists speculated that the nerves had a trophic function—that is, they would directly supply nutrients to body tissues—so it followed that a disturbance of a spinal nerve could materially weaken the organ it supplied.[48]

The faculty also seized upon the principle of "stimulation and inhibition" as advanced by C. E. Brown-Sequard (1817-94). In animal experiments he had discovered that a transverse sectioning of one lateral half of the base of the brain would be followed by augmentation of the motor properties in front of the cut, and by inhibition on the opposite side. A stimulus weaker than normal would then be sufficient to produce an effect in the first case, while a stronger stimulus would be necessary in the latter. This meant that an "irritation" of a given nerve not only could reduce action at one distant part, it could also increase action in another.[49] Charles Hazzard, in his interpretation of Brown-Sequard's doctrine, believed that by putting physical pressure on "vaso-motor centers" along the spinal column the osteopath could return excessive or insufficient functional activity within an organ back to normal, independent of the actual cause. If, for example, a patient was suffering from a bad case of indigestion and there was no discoverable disturbance in segmentally related vertebrae, one could nevertheless relieve the condition by treating the relevant centers.[50]

In addition to finding scientific evidence supporting Still's theory, the faculty also undertook the equally important task of making his ideas conform to established scientific facts, most notably the role of germs. From 1876, when Robert Koch (1843-1910) isolated the bacteria responsible for anthrax, to the dawn of the twentieth century, the microorganisms causing fourteen different afflictions of mankind were positively identified.[51] How could this be reconciled with the doctrine that anatomical misplacement was the major cause of disease? Similarly, what possible benefit could manipulating the spine have in treating infectious disorders? Still preferred to ignore the contradiction. "I believe but very little of the germ theory," he once declared, "and care much less."[52] All he seemed to admit to was their potential danger in open wounds.

His faculty, however, preferred to face the problem more directly. Each of them accepted the existence and etiological role of microorganisms. At the same time, Carl McConnell and the Littlejohns argued that while bacteriology seemed to undermine part of Still's original theory, its sister field, immunology, clearly supported him. Germs, they hypothesized, may be the active cause of disease, but spinal displacements, or what were now being called spinal "lesions," could be predisposing causes. If, as they believed, these structural lesions produced derangement of physiologic functions, it would follow that in their presence the body would automatically be put into a state of lowered resistance. Thus correcting lesions shortly after they occurred would lessen the likelihood of germs gaining a foothold in the body. By correcting lesions after infection had struck, the body's natural defenses could then more effectively respond to the invaders. Under these assumptions, osteopathic procedures seemed entirely applicable.[53]

Though he was at times disappointed and angry with his faculty because they sought to integrate the ideas of medical writers into their teachings,

Still did not seriously interfere.[54] As a result, their contribution to the future course of the profession was assured. While they had no appreciable effect on the number of patients and students coming to the Missouri Mecca, they laid the groundwork for building osteopathy upon an intellectual base broader than the one Still was capable of constructing himself.

# CHAPTER THREE

# In the Field

Although a few of Still's early graduates remained in Kirksville to serve as assistants in the infirmary, the majority went out into the field to establish their own private practices. A directory published in 1900 listing 717 graduates shows 121 (16.8 percent) residing in Missouri; 84 (11.7 percent) in Iowa; 83 (11.7 percent) in Illinois; 48 (6.6 percent) in Ohio; 32 (4.4 percent) in Pennsylvania; 31 (4.3 percent) in New York; and 30 (4.2 percent) in both Indiana and Tennessee respectively, with the rest scattered throughout thirty-five other states and territories.[1] Some returned to their home towns to begin work, while others were recruited by well-to-do patients who hired the new practitioners to accompany them back to their city of origin to continue the treatment. Under this sponsorship the osteopath was formally introduced to the entire community.

## Establishing a Practice

The most important task for the freshly settled D.O. was to create a favorable impression on the townspeople. The system was new and in many areas unheard of. Often the term *osteopathy* was a handicap; quite a few prospective patients took it to mean that D.O.'s thought all ailments were due to diseased bones or only treated fractures and dislocations. While in Kirksville, a few students recognized the potential problem and pleaded with Still to change the name. He remained adamant. "I don't care what Greek scholars say," he bristled, "I want to call my boy osteopathy."[2]

In their advertisements in local papers or in printed brochures and journals, D.O.'s explained that osteopathy was a totally original and independent system of health care. Several pointed out that it had "nothing in common with faith cure, Christian Science, spiritualism, hypnotism, magnetic healing, Swedish Movements, mental science, or massage."[3] Many in their audience, however, remained skeptical. All of these as well as other systems could involve, as did osteopathy, the "laying on of hands." Therese Cluett, D.O., of Cleveland, found that this led to much misunderstanding:

A lady entered my office and asked if I was a theosophist. I said, "No madam, I am an osteopathist." "Oh well," she replied, "It's all the same thing." Then it took me fully an hour to explain the difference between theosophy and osteopathy. On another occasion, I was approached with the question "Are you a Christian? because I don't want to take treatment from anyone who is not a Christian." This fairly caught my breath. . . . I asked her if she had put the same question to [her last physician] that she had put to me. She replied that she had not. It took me another hour to explain the difference between osteopathy and Christianity. For one patient I have to insulate the table, as they think this is some form of magnetic treatment. The next patient spies the insulators (as I had forgotten to remove them) and then there is trouble, as this patient won't have anything along that line of business.[4]

Cluett's problem was shared by Herbert Bernard, D.O., who noted, "When I first came to Detroit, a woman telephoned me asking what price I charged to pray for people. Another one looked all over one of my operating tables trying to find the electric wires that he thought were hidden. . . . Quick results were dangerous in those days, as the patients would think there had been some rabbit's foot business worked upon them. They were afraid to tell of their relief . . . thinking people would take them for faith-cure followers."[5]

In explaining their system and differentiating it from others, many osteopaths told their patients that they alone could be considered "anatomical engineers." Only D.O.'s knew where every bone, muscle, nerve, or blood vessel should be and what significance each held in the maintenance or restoration of health. Several of them published descriptions that were eloquently worded and simple to understand. If one accepted the metaphor of man as a machine, the osteopath's logic made sense. As a violin or engine needed tuning or adjustment every so often, so also did the human body.

On the other hand, a good number of practitioners preferred the hard-sell approach, which, though less dignified, was nonetheless successful in drawing attention. "Osteopathy," said one appeal, "deserves your patronage because it has demonstrated its ability to do all medicine can do and much more. Many are the diseases entirely beyond the reach of the medical attendant that promptly surrender to the ability and the knowledge of the osteopath. In other words, there is not a single thing that medical men can surpass osteopaths in except . . . malpractice or killing people."[6]

Quite a few D.O.'s published lists of the diseases that they claimed to be especially successful in treating. A typical list included "headache, granulated eyelids, deafness, dripping eyes, dizziness, pterygium, polyps of the nose, catarrh, constipation, torpid liver, gall stones, neuralgia of the stomach and bowels, dysentery, flux, piles, fistula, irregularities of the heart, kidney diseases, female diseases, rheumatism and neuralgia of all parts, atrophy of the limbs, paralysis, locomotor ataxia, varicose veins, milk leg eczema, nervous prostration, hip joint disease, curvature of the spine, etc."[7] Some placed recovery percentages next to disorders, such as one list, which reported: sleeplessness, 95 percent; back pain, 90 percent; stomach trouble, 75 percent; dropsy, 65 percent; withered limbs, 60 percent; deafness, 55 percent; and cancer, 30 percent.[8] Others gave overall figures. "We cure about eight-five percent of the cases we take," declared one infirmary, "benefit ninety-five percent, and fail on five percent."[9]

Another advertising method was the testimonial. Gratified patients would give the practitioner permission to publish flattering letters they had written. In defending this approach, the Matthews and Hook Infirmary declared, "Osteopathy is a great discovery. Its theory is most reasonable. But it has a practical side as well as a reasonable theory. And while it is perfectly proper to give its principles, its scientific basis, and speak in general terms of what it can do, it is also eminently necessary to take evidence and hear testimony from those who have tried it. . . . The question that the world asks is 'Does it work?' Osteopathy works. And for the benefit of those who wish to investigate we shall give from time to time the names and addresses of some who have thoroughly tested it."[10]

Most of the individuals who patronized the early D.O.'s suffered from chronic complaints similar to those found among patrons of the Missouri Mecca. "During our twenty months practice in Nashville," Dr. J. R. Schackleford noted, "we have had many cases of interest, some of whom had gone the rounds of the medical profession, patent medicine, sanitariums, springs, mountains, sea shore, and various other devices and places for relief. Many who came said to us 'We have tried everything else and now we are willing to try osteopathy.' This is the rule in most cases, but whether we are the first or last makes but little difference to us so [long as] we get the desired results."[11] Though some of the clinic reports sent into the *Journal of Osteopathy* concerned acute infectious disorders, these represented a minor portion of the average osteopathic workload. As W. L. Riggs, D.O., wrote, "The idea is generally prevalent among the laity, wherever osteopathy is known, that the science is peculiarly adapted to longstanding and chronic cases, but that its results are too slow to counter-act the rapid processes which follow the conditions prevailing in what are commonly called acute diseases."[12]

Patients were generally told that quick cures were the exception rather than the rule. Most D.O.'s agreed with Dr. A. L. Evans, who observed:

The over sanguine osteopath who advertises, writes, and talks constantly about cases that are remarkable for the rapidity with which they have yielded to osteopathic treatment does himself and the profession an injustice. People are led to expect miracles. . . . It is wise to explain to them that it will take time to eliminate poisonous drugs from their system and to induce healthy normal action in torpid organs that have long been dependent upon extraneous stimulation. It is far better to impress this upon them than to tell wonderful stories—no matter how true—of marvelous cures effected in one or two treatments. By the latter method the patient is led to expect the same results in his own case and may be disappointed, for nature, though sure, is sometimes slow. If, on the other hand, more is accomplished than promised, osteopathy has won a friend that will never falter in allegiance to our system.[13]

To encourage this type of thinking, D.O.'s generally billed their patients by the month, charging the standard fee for four weeks of treatment of twenty-five dollars. If the client's condition required an extended period, a sliding scale of charges was often worked out.

One problem generated by this arrangement was that patients expected as many sessions within the month as possible, regardless of their ailment. As a result, it became a matter of custom to administer three treatments per week per client. Therese Cluett wrote of one supplicant who wanted "a treatment 'everyday' as Mrs. So-and-so goes to Dr. So-and-so and he gives a treatment 'everyday.' I say 'All right' knowing well it is only a question of time until she will beg off. In a week the patient is so prostrated by the frequent treatment that she is glad to admit she cannot stand so much osteopathy. It is all I can do to get her three times a week which is as much as anyone can stand without becoming debilitated."[14] Since each of these encounters could last up to one hour, fatigue on the part of the patient as well as the practitioner can be clearly imagined.

Of the early D.O.'s in the field who contributed letters to the *Journal of Osteopathy* and other periodicals, almost all boasted that they were making a good living. In 1898 Joseph Sullivan, D.O., declared "Osteopathy in Chicago is on the high road to success. We are treating more people now than at any time during '97 and our results are most gratifying." Drs. F. W. and Mrs. Hannah noted, "Our patients now number three score of the leading people of Detroit and vicinity including representatives from almost every profession and avenue of business."[15] Drs. Mason Pressly and O. J. Snyder of Philadelphia claimed, "Within so short a time as a year . . . our books show that we are treating considerably over a hundred patients every month."[16] In explaining the osteopath's success, A. L. Evans listed several major factors: First, the theory of osteopathy was a rational and common-sense one; there was nothing "vague, mysterious, or occult about it." Second was the plain and reasonable plan of charges, "a system whereby the patient is enabled to tell approximately what it is going to cost him to regain his health." Third, manipulation was much more palatable to the patient than medicine or surgery: "If osteopathy did nothing but abolish

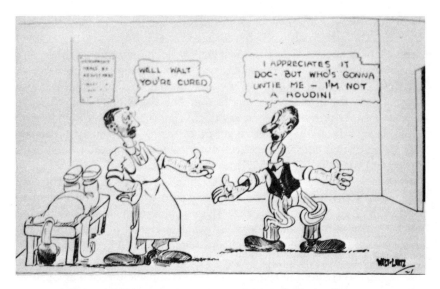

*Cartoonist Walter Lantz's view of osteopathic treatment (1921)*

experimental doses of poisonous drugs and curtail the number of blood operations it would be worthy of the gratitude of countless sufferers." And finally, Evans argued, "nothing succeeds like success. It is results that tell."[17]

Such missives of self-congratulation did not give a complete accounting of the situation, however. Each issue of the *Journal* would also contain notices by many D.O.'s of a change of address, often from town to town. For them, osteopathy was not a sure-paying proposition, and not a few dropped out of practice altogether.[18] In many instances the business failure of the osteopath was due to public apathy; in others, an inability to impress his or her clientele was to blame. For some, it was a matter of the local M.D.'s employing existing medical licensing acts to drive them out before they had a chance to get settled in.

### Legal Struggles

The posture of the orthodox physician towards the osteopath varied considerably. Some regarded the practitioner as a harmless quack whose clientele would patronize any new healer who happened to arrive in town. A few thought that their "rubbing" might be indicated in selected cases and would even refer an occasional patient or two. Most often, the M.D.'s' response was shaped by the behavior of the D.O. If the latter went quietly about his business there was usually a small chance of confrontation. However, the osteopath who arrived in town with much fanfare, making extravagant claims regarding his own skill while intimating that the M.D.'s were in league with the undertakers, was simply asking to be prosecuted. Whenever arrests did take place, the D.O.'s would maintain that jealousy and fear were the prime motivating factors. Once they had begun to prove they were superior doctors, their argument ran, the M.D.'s in self-defense would have to do all they could to get rid of them. While many did depart after being hauled before the courts, other osteopaths stayed to fight, and in the great majority of instances they managed to win.

The first legal action regarding a D.O. in the field appears to be the case of Charles Still (1865-1955), the founder's son, who had been invited to practice in Red Wing, Minnesota. When he arrived in 1893 he found himself in the midst of an epidemic of what had been diagnosed by local doctors as diphtheria. Though his experience to date had been with chronic disorders, Still was soon called upon to treat a victim. After his patient made a rapid recovery following conscientious applications of manipulative treatments to the neck, shoulders, and head, Still was asked to care for upwards of seventy children with reportedly only one fatality as a result. The State Board of Health, despite his apparent success, authorized his arrest for practicing without a license. By the time the case came up for trial Still's work had generated such considerable public support that the M.D. who initiated the suit decided not to make an appearance, and the matter was dropped.[19]

Audrey C. Moore, D.O., a graduate of the American School of Osteopathy's second class, was practicing in Macon, Illinois, when he was jailed on a similar charge. In his defense, Moore produced patients who testified that he had benefited or cured them when their M.D. had given up hope. "After examining a number of my witnesses," he recalled, "none of whom had seen any medicines used, and all of whom felt better after treatment, the justice said from the bench that the people seemed to want to try this new humbug, so he would discharge the prisoner."[20]

A few D.O.'s were even emboldened to initiate legal action against the M.D.'s. In 1898 Harry Nelson, D.O., who had been practicing in Louisville for about a year, became tired of the threats issued by the Kentucky Board of Health that he had better either leave town or prepare himself for incarceration. In his suit, Nelson demanded that the board examine and license him or else cease and desist. When the matter came to trial Nelson's patients testified on his behalf; but unlike in the Moore case, the presiding judge was not impressed. Instead he listened to John McCormack, M.D., of the American Medical Association, who maintained that "to license Dr. Nelson would be dangerous to the health, limbs, and lives of those citizens who might be treated by him in most instances." Though he lost this round, Nelson would not give up his fight. The following year he brought his case to the court of appeals, which reversed the original decision and granted a permanent injunction against the board from preventing any D.O. from engaging in his profession. "So long as he confines himself to osteopathy, without the use of medicine or surgical appliances," the court ruled, "he violates no law and appellee should not molest him."[21]

What constituted the practice of medicine became the primary legal point at issue in most of the state courts that entertained such suits. M.D. representatives argued that *medicine* as found in the various healing arts statutes should be construed in its widest possible sense, while the D.O.'s maintained that it meant the practice of administering drugs—and nothing more. In Alabama the state supreme court took the side of the M.D.'s, deciding "It is made entirely clear both by definitions and history that the word medicine has a technical meaning, is a technical art or science, and as a science the practitioners of it are not simply those who prescribe drugs, or other medical substances as remedial agents, but that it is broad enough to include all persons who diagnose disease and prescribe or apply any therapeutic agent for its cure."[22] However, only the Nebraska judiciary agreed. All other high courts ruling before 1904—Colorado, New York, North Carolina, Mississippi, Virginia, Ohio, and New Jersey—concurred with Kentucky that the concept should be narrowly interpreted.[23] "In forbidding an unlicensed person to apply any drug or medicine for remedial purposes," said the New Jersey high court, "the legislature plainly contemplated the use of something other than the natural facilities of the actor; some extraneous substance."[24]

In addition to their judicial struggles, both the M.D.'s and D.O.'s traveled legislative avenues, appearing before a number of state legislatures to present their respective cases; the former sought specifically to outlaw the new system, while the latter wished to establish standards governing its practice. The first successful effort by the D.O.'s came in Vermont. Physicians in and nearby the town of Chelsea had become upset over the activities of Dr. George Helmer, who had established an osteopathic infirmary there in 1895. As Helmer's clientele grew the M.D.'s complained to the state's attorney that the new healer was a public menace who preyed upon the weak-minded. Since several of the official's friends were among those being treated, their demands for prosecution were not looked upon favorably. This prompted the Vermont Medical Association to call upon the legislature for relief. Apprised of this, Helmer temporarily moved his offices to the capital to fight. While he was there, several lawmakers with chronic health problems decided to find out for themselves the relative merits of osteopathy by willingly submitting to his treatments. A number of them, including the lieutenant governor, were most pleased. As a consequence the legislature decided to throw out the medical society's bill, substituting and passing one giving any graduate of the American School of Osteopathy the right "to practice their art of healing in the state."[25]

Next in line to regulate the new system was North Dakota. Though D.O.'s were involved in this lobbying effort, the battle was primarily waged by a patient, Helen DeLenderecie, the wife of "the merchant prince of Fargo." Her motivation was well expressed in a letter she wrote to the *Journal of Osteopathy:*

> In the fall of 1895, a lump appeared in my right breast. Our family physician advised its immediate removal assuring me that nothing but the knife could remedy the evil, and stating that it would soon assume a malignant form if not removed without delay. Knowing him to be a fine surgeon as well as a physician, I placed myself in his hands and submitted to an operation whereby my entire breast was removed. It was a great shock to my nervous system, and I had not recovered from it, when the same trouble appeared in my left breast. I had heard meantime of osteopathy and resolved to try it before again submitting to the knife. . . . I went to Kirksville and was completely cured in six weeks time. My own eyes saw and my own hands felt the obstruction that caused the trouble in both cases, and I knew very well that the knife was never necessary. . . . Osteopathy has clearly proven its right to recognition in the healing of cases heretofore declared only curable by the knife, and it is only right that its supporters should sustain its claim.[26]

When the bill came up for a vote in the senate, DeLenderecie was given the unusual privilege of speaking to the entire body in its support. After hearing her dramatic story and her rebuttals of some of the arguments put forward by the M.D.'s, the legislature passed the measure, and the governor, another osteopathic patient, happily signed it.[27]

Though subsequent battles were not all so easily won, and in many cases initial osteopathic efforts were rebuffed because of the M.D.'s' lobbying efforts, by 1901 thirteen additional states—Missouri (1897), Michigan (1897), Iowa (1898), South Dakota (1899), Illinois (1899), Tennessee (1899), Montana (1901), Kansas (1901), California (1901), Indiana (1901), Nebraska (1901), Wisconsin (1901), and Connecticut (1901)—had established laws regulating the practice of the new system.[28] Many orthodox physicians had first thought osteopathy only a fad, but it became increasingly apparent to them that the actions of most courts and legislatures were encouraging its growth and subsequent institutionalization.[29] At the turn of the century, when the American Medical Association was making considerable progress in eliminating the homeopathic and eclectic schools through a process of absorption, here was yet another competitor threatening to take the M.D.'s' place.[30]

## Other Schools

While the fight in the courts and legislatures was in progress, a number of Still's graduates were forming their own colleges. The first were the National School of Osteopathy (1895) of Kansas City; the Pacific College of Osteopathy (1896) of Los Angeles; and the Northern Institute of Osteopathy (1896) of Minneapolis. Within a few years the products of these schools, as well as of the American School of Osteopathy, established colleges in Boston, Philadelphia, San Francisco, Des Moines, Milwaukee, Chicago, Denver, and in smaller cities such as Wilkes-Barre, Pennsylvania; Ottawa, Kansas; Franklin, Kentucky; Fargo, North Dakota; Keokuk, Iowa; and Quincy, Illinois. Most of these institutions grew out of existing infirmaries where some clients, seeing and experiencing the benefits of osteopathy first hand, were anxious to become practitioners themselves. Instead of sending them to Kirksville, diplomates with an eye toward supplementing their income were quite willing to organize their own programs. By 1904, of the estimated four thousand D.O.'s in practice, approximately one-half were graduates of these other schools.[31]

Initially the physical plants of these colleges consisted of a small suite of rooms in an office building or a converted private residence. Since the first few classes were small, such facilities were seen by their proprietors as more than adequate. Entrance standards were nominal. While a number of catalogs called for a high school diploma, students lacking one found little difficulty in gaining admittance, provided they were able to pay their fee in advance. Tuition was generally set at the American School of Osteopathy's original figure of five hundred dollars for the complete course, but because of competition it was soon lowered to a more reasonable three hundred to three hundred fifty dollars, which in turn increased the number of matriculants.

At first there was no common standard relating to the length and breadth of the course. Some colleges, following the American School, limited their instruction to several months of anatomy, osteopathic diagnosis, and therapy, while others took it upon themselves to increase the time necessary for graduation as well as the number of subjects covered. Indeed, the Pacific College was the first to adopt a curriculum consisting of four terms of five months each which included broad basic science instruction.[32] When Still followed suit, months later, most of the others decided to go along.

The faculty of these schools were generally composed of from three to ten professors, depending on the number of students enrolled. In some cases more than one-half of the instructors did not possess a D.O. degree or have any previous osteopathic training. M.D.'s who wanted to learn something of their techniques as an adjunct to their own practice were pressed into teaching some subjects in lieu of part or the whole of their tuition fee. In almost all cases M.D.'s, whether they served on the faculty or not, were automatically given advanced standing, allowing them to complete the requirements for their diploma in half the normal time.[33]

The equipment in these institutions varied markedly. Where the American School, the Des Moines School, and the Pacific College were able to move quickly into large, spacious facilities and furnish their laboratories with microscopes, dissecting and chemical analysis kits, as well as the newly invented x-ray machine, many others seem to have gotten along with a treatment table, a skeleton, and a few wall charts.[34]

In urging prospective students to enroll, each catalog made osteopathy appear as a great calling and focused on the inner satisfaction one could expect by healing people in this "natural drugless way." However, if this was not sufficient motivation, there was always the appeal to one's mercenary interest. "The experience of graduates of osteopathy, who are now practicing in various parts of the country," claimed the Des Moines College, "demonstrates conclusively that there is no profession at this time in existence where a young man or woman can earn money so rapidly and successfully as in the practice of osteopathy. We have data in our office to show that good, scientific graduates of osteopathy can go out and earn from $250 to $500 per month, and in some cases their earnings reach as high as $800 a month."[35] The Northern School was even more encouraging, declaring, "Osteopathy is the business opportunity of one's life time. There is increasing demand for it. No student properly equipped has made a failure of it. Individuals are making in cash from $500 to $1,000 per month. We know men who couldn't earn $1,000 a year who are now making $1,000 per month."[36]

Where there might be as many as a dozen M.D.'s in a small community, one argument ran, there would be a single D.O. who, after he cured but a few of his counterpart's failures, would be swamped with more business than he could handle. An early catalog of the Philadelphia College observed, "There are not yet 400 osteopaths in the country, with a population of 75,000,000. The supply is short . . . the demand is great and there is no competition. This opens up a highway to success."[37] Correspondingly, the Atlantic School in Wilkes-Barre noted, "Fifty or one hundred years hence the profession will be crowded, but it will not be while we live. Those first in any field are the ones that reap the harvest—not the gleaners."[38]

Special appeals were directed at prospective female candidates. Since they were then denied entrance to all but a handful of regular medical schools, here was an alternative method of becoming a doctor. "The science of osteopathy appeals to women who desire a noble, uplifting work," the Pacific College reasoned. "A woman whose natural inclination is toward the benefit and assistance of the less fortunate of human kind, and who desires to allay herself with some work that while acting constantly as a moral uplift, will yet be in an agreeable and rapid way place her peculiarly above all concern for the future, has the basis furnished her in osteopathy."[39] Such inducements were apparently quite successful, since approximately one-fifth of all graduates of osteopathic schools before 1910 were women.[40]

Each college naturally pointed to itself as the most advantageous institution in which to learn to become an osteopath. In addition to citing the alleged quality of their respective facilities, equipment, and staff, many focused on the environmental conditions of the city in which their school was located. "Franklin," said the Southern School, "is a noted health resort having several mineral wells whose properties are seldom excelled."[41] Similarly, the Pacific College declared Los Angeles to be "the best place in the world to study hard and maintain one's bodily vigor."[42] The Des Moines College even made a contrast between its town and the Missouri Mecca, claiming its "streets are well improved and the climate is exceptionally healthy," while Kirksville, because of supposedly poor sanitary conditions, "was rapidly becoming a hotbed for typhoid and malarial fever."[43]

Relations between these new colleges and the American School of Osteopathy were at best correct and at worst openly hostile. Still believed that few if any of his early graduates had either the training or the practical experience to teach osteopathy on their own; that their institutions, for the most part, did not match the standards of the American School of Osteopathy; and finally, since some of them were situated within a few hundred miles of Kirksville, that they were in open competition for students who should rightfully be his.

The American School of Osteopathy declared war on the National School in nearby Kansas City almost from its inception. The National School, headed by Elmer and Helen Barber, two graduates of the American School's second class, had a regular course of instruction that was somewhat briefer than the one found at the parent institution, and it was rumored that its diplomas could be bought for a price. Elmer wrote the first book ever published on osteopathy, and in it he claimed that Still was wrong on a number of important theoretical issues, and that anyone could learn to treat common ailments manipulatively with his text as the only necessary aid.[44] Not surprisingly, M.D. groups found Barber's work a most useful illustration of their contention that osteopathy was a fraud.

As a result of these goings-on, Still and his associates were placed on the defensive; they did all they could to dissociate themselves from and repudiate the Barbers, Elmer's book, and the National School. William Smith, who had entered private practice for a time after teaching the first class and who had thus never met the twosome, was dispatched to Kansas

City to determine whether they were complying with the new state law that required a college to give twenty months of personal instruction before awarding a diploma.[45] Meeting Elmer under an assumed name, Smith identified himself as an M.D. who knew all about osteopathy though he did not have the benefit of a D.O. degree. Barber, in turn, offered to issue him one on the spot for $150, a sum Smith agreed to and then paid. He next stopped at the attorney general's office, where he presented the bogus diploma and related the facts of the case, all of which led to the Barbers' indictment. Although he found the pair guilty of violating the new statute, the judge refused to accede to the prosecutor's demand that their charter be revoked, finding that Smith's actual medical and osteopathic education mitigated the seriousness of the offense. After paying a small fine, the Barbers continued as before. Only in 1900, when their operation proved to be unprofitable, did they voluntarily decide to close their doors, but not before bestowing degrees on at least fifty individuals, some of whom established their own diploma mills, such as Noe's College of Osteopathy in San Francisco and Payne's College of Osteopathy and Optics in Ottawa, Kansas.[46]

Even more galling to Still than the Barber's institution was the Columbian School of Osteopathy, located almost across the street from the American School and run by a former associate, Marcus Ward (1849-1929). Brought to Kirksville on a stretcher in 1890, Ward looked to Still for relief from a severe asthmatic condition. After he was restored to health, Ward entered into a business arrangement with his benefactor to learn his methods. Still later took him on as one of his assistants in the infirmary, and when Still established the American School of Osteopathy in 1892 Ward became a major stockholder and served as vice-president under the first charter. Within months after the college opened, however, the two had a falling out, and as a result Ward left town. He eventually relocated in Ohio, enrolling in the medical department of the University of Cincinnati; after obtaining his M.D. degree there in 1897, he moved back to Kirksville. There, with the help of local businessmen who believed the town was large enough for two osteopathic institutions, he established the Columbian School.[47]

In his advertising Ward declared himself the "co-founder of osteopathy" and claimed to have been working along the same lines as Still since 1862, when he was thirteen years old. He also called himself the sole originator of what he named "True Osteopathy," which was the combination of *materia medica,* surgery, and manipulation. The use of all three therapeutic modalities, said Ward, would reestablish the "true" approach to healing as practiced by the Ancient Greeks. Columbian students were therefore taught the principles of drug therapy along with other subjects now found in the expanded American School of Osteopathy curriculum. After they completed their twenty-month course and received the D.O. degree they could enroll for another year of medical and surgical training, upon completion of which they would be granted the M.D.[48]

Still wisely decided not to dignify Ward's inflated claim of being the co-discoverer. This he left to his friends and associates.[49] He did, however, sharply lash out at Ward's inclusion of *materia medica* in his curriculum. "Every man and woman sick and tired of drugs, opiates, stimulants, laxatives, and purgatives has turned with longing eyes to this rainbow of hope [Kirksville]," he thundered, "and yet these medical osteopaths are trying to paint this rainbow with calomel and perfume it with whiskey." Ward's college, he opined, was a mongrel institution that, like the bat, is "neither bird nor beast." Anyone who pays his money into it "gets neither medicine nor osteopathy, but a smattering, enough to make a first class quack."[50]

In its first two years of operation, the Columbian School attracted a fair number of matriculants; however, internal disputes between Ward and his backers would thereafter rack the college, and the institution closed in 1901 after graduating perhaps as many as seventy individuals. Once again the "co-founder" left town, eventually settling in California, where for the next quarter-century he practiced in relative obscurity.[51] Though ostracized from the movement and quickly forgotten, Ward, with his efforts at fully integrating drug therapy into the osteopathic system, was a harbinger of battles to come.

# CHAPTER FOUR

# *Structure and Function*

With the movement rapidly growing, many D.O.'s thought it desirable to coordinate their efforts and activities. In February of 1897, a small group of American School of Osteopathy alumni met in Kirksville and decided to establish a national organization for this purpose. Graduates of other schools were then invited to take part in the planning, and by April they collectively launched the American Association for the Advancement of Osteopathy, which was renamed and restructured as the American Osteopathic Association (AOA) four years later.[1]

The officers of the AOA under its 1901 constitution included a president, two vice-presidents, a secretary, and a treasurer, all chosen for a twelve-month period of service, and a Board of Trustees whose members were appointed for staggered three-year terms. Members of the board were charged with responsibility for the day-to-day affairs of the association, while the general membership—in reality only those opting to attend the annual convention—elected all officers, including the board, and decided questions of policy.[2] As the number of AOA members rose, this last feature of the system proved unwieldy, prompting those participating in the 1909 convention to enlarge the board from eleven to seventeen members and invest it with virtually complete control over policy issues.[3] In 1919 a dual form of central government was restored when a House of Delegates was created based on the proportional number of state members. These representatives, who were chosen by their respective divisional societies, thereafter selected all other national office-holders and acted as the business body of the association during its annual week-long meetings.[4]

From its inception, the AOA actively worked to secure the conditions necessary for the movement to obtain professional recognition. With regard to autonomy, it fought for independent boards of registration and examination; on the academic front, it both significantly lengthened the standard course of undergraduate training and supported ongoing research projects; and in terms of socioeconomic status, it championed a code of ethics while combatting the growth of impostors and imitators.

## The Independent Board

At the turn of the century a majority of states were without a specific law governing osteopathy, and in several of the states with such a law, the legal position of the D.O. was hardly improved as a consequence. Early lobbying campaigns had usually been conducted by individuals speaking for only one segment of the emerging movement, leading to situations such as that in Vermont, which had extended practice rights only to graduates of the American School.[5] In other states diverse osteopathic factions had appeared before the legislatures with varying recommendations. This lack of unanimity often resulted in a poorly constructed compromise or no law at all.

Several of the early acts placed the regulation of osteopathy under the jurisdiction of existing state medical boards. In some cases a D.O. was added to these agencies; in others no representation was granted. Although osteopaths would be examined alongside M.D.'s, taking the same written tests in such subjects as anatomy, physiology, and chemistry, they were exempted from answering questions concerning *materia medica* or therapeutics. In a few states this arrangement seemed to work out satisfactorily for the D.O.'s, as they found they could do nearly as well as the allopaths in passing examinations and becoming licensed. However, before other similarly constituted boards this did not occur, and in certain instances M.D. officials prevented any comparison between the two groups whatsoever. In Iowa, for example, the legislature granted the medical board the power of accrediting osteopathic schools, with only graduates from approved institutions becoming eligible for licensure. After a cursory look at their catalogs, the board rejected all of the colleges, thereby preventing any D.O. from legitimately practicing in the state and thus circumventing the intent of the lawmakers.[6]

In 1901 the AOA created a permanent Committee on Legislation in order to insure the passage of favorable laws. Toward this end, the committee devised a standard model bill for every state whose chief feature was the establishment of independent boards of osteopathic examination and registration. According to this proposal, each divisional association would nominate a long list of candidates from which the governor of the state would choose five to serve as members. These individuals, once they had been appointed, would be responsible for testing candidates, negotiating reciprocity agreements with other boards, and disciplining errant practitioners.[7] With the AOA trustees giving their strong backing to the idea, the committee began overseeing the lobbying efforts of the divisional societies. Frequently the societies faced an especially hard struggle. When medical practice arts were reintroduced in the 1870s and 1880s, several states granted the allopaths, homeopaths, and eclectics separate boards.

This arrangement was sometimes difficult to administer and was often plagued by licensing inequities. However, by abolishing this system, and placing representatives of each sect upon a single board where they kept a watchful eye on one another, some legislatures had found that these problems were less likely to occur. As a consequence of this experience, lawmakers, while quite willing to grant the osteopaths basic legal rights, were reluctant to furnish them with the means of self-regulation.[8]

In appealing to those who either were undecided on the issue or saw no need for independent boards, Arthur Hildreth, D.O. (1863-1941), the first chairman of the Committee on Legislation, hastened to argue:

> There has never been one single voice raised against osteopathy except by men of other medical schools. Every inch of progress made by our profession since its discovery has been contested by them. We have been looked down upon, criticized, ridiculed, called "faddists," "masseurs" and everything but gentlemen. And now when securing recognition by law, should we secure representation from existing Boards of Examination and Registration, we should have to do so against their protest and through the influence of our many, many, good friends. And after securing representation upon their boards, what is our position? Are we loved any more by them? No, we are still at a disadvantage because they overwhelm us in numbers and ours being unwelcome company, we need not expect many favors. Certainly we shall receive no help to reach out and grasp greater and better things such as must and will come to us with the right kind of encouragement and conditions.[9]

This line of reasoning became increasingly influential over the years, particularly where elected officials became convinced that discrimination by M.D. boards did in fact take place. In 1913, of the thirty-nine states that had passed osteopathic practice laws, seventeen provided for independent boards. Ten years later, these figures rose to forty-six and twenty-seven respectively.[10] Furthermore, even in many of those states whose legislatures refused to accede to all D.O. requests, bills were enacted recognizing the AOA as the sole accrediting agency of osteopathic colleges, thereby preventing prejudicial actions by M.D. boards. Accordingly, the profession won for itself a considerable degree of autonomy and legal security.

### Lengthening the Course

The first group within the movement that attempted to set common educational requirements was the Associated Colleges of Osteopathy (ACO), founded in 1898 and composed of most of the legitimate schools. In fact, from the time of the ACO's formation, eligibility for membership in the AOA was predicated on being a graduate of an ACO-affiliated institution.[11] The Associated Colleges was created in part to remove the ill feelings the schools bore towards each other because of their aggressive competition for matriculants. Certain activities then engaged in—such as cutting tuition, stealing students, and shortening the time necessary to earn a diploma—were clearly working to their mutual detriment. To stop these practices, each member of the ACO pledged to adhere to clear guidelines covering admissions, attendance, tuition, transfers, advertising methods, and a mandatory two-year course.[12] Nevertheless, despite their promises, some of the colleges continued in these prohibited practices, which only engendered further suspicion and distrust. As it became obvious that the schools could not effectively regulate themselves, the AOA in 1901 ruled that henceforth it would be the final arbiter in approving the colleges from which its own members would originate, thus in effect making the association the primary authority for establishing and maintaining standards.[13]

Looking at the state of osteopathic education at this juncture, leaders of the profession were convinced that major improvements were called for. One of the critical areas of concern was the length of time needed to train and graduate D.O.'s. Certainly the two-year curriculum of twenty months looked meager beside the four-year, thirty-six-month program offered by almost all the allopathic institutions. As Wilfred Harris, D.O., head of the Massachusetts school, argued, "The twenty month course is too brief. However clever the student, he cannot by any process of mental gymnastics, transplant himself with such suddenness from one field of thought and activity to another."[14] In 1902 the newly organized AOA Committee on Education issued a report urging the rapid establishment of a three-year course and the introduction of a four-year curriculum as soon as practicable.[15] According to its chairman, C.M.T. Hulett, this "would give time for more exhaustive work in many subjects now too much abridged; would make possible a substitution of the laboratory for the lecture, in many cases, and permit good laboratory work being made better."[16]

Not all D.O.'s, however, saw matters in this light. Some believed that laboratory instruction was relatively unimportant. Others took the self-serving position that in adding one year and eventually another to the course, the profession would be declaring all previous graduates inferior or unqualified. This argument was skillfully answered by J. Martin Littlejohn, who along with his brothers had left Kirksville in 1900 to establish a school in Chicago. "The question is often asked did not our earlier graduates get along on much less time? Yes; but none have felt more than they the handicap that meant," he declared. "We do not mean they have not succeeded. They did succeed, but theirs was a struggle to evolve their knowledge as they advanced. To the busy practitioner, this is no easy matter."[17]

In 1903 the AOA and ACO jointly sponsored the first on-site survey of the schools. Chosen as inspector was Eamons R. Booth (1851-1934), who before becoming a D.O. had earned a Ph.D. from Wooster College and had taught at Washington University in St. Louis. In his report to the profession, Booth confirmed what others had already claimed in regard to the depth of preparation possible under the existing curriculum. His findings and recommendations helped to sway the undecided; the AOA voted to require that all colleges inaugurate a compulsory three-year, twenty-seven-month course by September, 1904.[18]

A number of schools harbored great reservations concerning this policy, fearing a sudden drop in matriculants. Three early members of the ACO — the Milwaukee College (1898-1901), the Northern Institute of Minneapolis (1896-1902), and the Northwestern College at Fargo (1898-1903) — had all recently folded primarily because of insufficient enrollment. The new requirement might accelerate this trend. Curiously, the greatest objections were raised by the most solvent of all. Charles Still claimed that all his father's assets were tied up in the American School of Osteopathy and that in the event of a disaster the "old doctor" would be ruined. The younger Still pleaded for an optional rather than a mandatory three-year course, but the plea was rejected by the AOA, which subsequently decided by a narrow margin to give Kirksville an additional twelve-month grace period.[19]

While the total number of osteopathic matriculants in the following decade did in fact markedly decline as predicted, some schools were more dramatically affected than others. Closing their doors were the Colorado College of Denver (1897-1904); the Atlantic School, first of Wilkes-Barre, Pennsylvania, later of Buffalo, New York (1898-1905); the Southern School of Franklin, Kentucky (1898-1907); and the California College of San Francisco (1898-1910). In 1914 two others, the Los Angeles and Pacific colleges, agreed to merge. As of 1915 there were only seven recognized D.O.-granting schools operating, located in Boston, Chicago, Des Moines, Kansas City, Kirksville, Los Angeles, and Philadelphia.

For most of these colleges the addition of the third year had unexpectedly worked to improve their financial situation, as the decrease in new matriculants was more than offset by the proportionately higher tuition fee each enrolled student paid. This led all of them to initiate an optional four-year course. In 1911 Philadelphia, spurred by recently enacted requirements for college registration in key states like New York, made the extra year compulsory for new matriculants.[20] It was soon joined by Chicago.[21] In 1914 the AOA Board of Trustees passed a resolution stipulating that the remainder of the colleges do the same no later than 1916.[22] Although some of the schools once again feared dire consequences because of this move, they realized they had no choice but to comply. By 1920 all graduates of approved osteopathic colleges had received a length of instruction equivalent to their M.D. counterparts.

## Scientific Publications and Research

In 1901 the AOA introduced the *Journal of the American Osteopathic Association* (*JAOA*), whose purpose was to inform members of organizational business and to advance scientific knowledge. Within two years the *JAOA* was being issued on a monthly basis with each edition consisting of approximately fifty pages. Its staff recognized that for the *JAOA* to become a truly professional publication, the quality of its articles on practice, particularly those based on actual case histories, would have to rise above the level then prevalent. As one prominent D.O. succinctly remarked:

> It has long been appreciated by the public fully as well as oursevles, that osteopathic clinic reports in the true sense of the word DO NOT EXIST. What we call clinic reports and print in our magazines are a hodge podge of "hot air" and personal advertising in which we grant each other the right to advance rhetorically each his or her own personal reputation just as much as possible. . . . When [in] issue after issue our papers print glowing reports of what we have all done, and at that over our own signatures, isn't it just a little likely that the conscientious enquirer will say "Well do these people ever admit failures? Do they know where they fail to cure?"[23]

In order to improve the quality of osteopathic case reporting, the AOA Committee on Publication in 1902 appointed Edythe Ashmore, D.O., of Detroit, to lead a campaign in which practitioners in the field would be encouraged to fill out and submit concise patient histories, the best of which would be published in sets of one hundred as a semiannual *JAOA* supplement. This effort, it was thought, not only would be good experience, but would also help to establish the D.O.'s' claims. Ashmore mailed out forms specifying the type of information needed, including client's age, sex, marital status, occupation, family history, prior treatment, symptoms, physical signs and diagnosis, what osteopathic lesions were present, the causes of disease other than lesions, and what urinalysis and other laboratory tests revealed. In terms of therapy, Ashmore requested descriptions of the specific manipulative technique employed, the length of treatment, and changes in method as the case progressed.[24]

The first series was published in 1904, the last in 1909.[25] In each installment cases were divided into eight broad disease classifications. Representation of given disorders did not always reflect the frequency of their appearance in a typical osteopathic practice; rather, many patient histories seem to have been selected on the basis of their value in demonstrating the allegedly wide applications of Still's approach. While most of these printed cases were described with the needless bluster, self-advertising, and harangues against the M.D.'s eliminated, serious problems remained. Only a small number of examples where manipulation was found to be ineffective were included. Though these supplements were not meant for patient distribution, most D.O.'s had no desire to appear as anything less than successful before their peers. Another difficulty was the obvious lack of consistency in diagnostic findings. In a given condition, for example, asthma, one D.O. would find lesions along the cervical spine, another in the dorsal area, while a third located them in the lumbar region; and each would announce positive results by manipulating only where the lesions were said to be.[26] With the M.D.'s charging that such lesions were imaginary and that osteopaths wrought their cures simply through suggestion, these seemingly conflicting reports would not help the D.O.'s in refuting their critics.

As this weakness became manifest, influential D.O.'s sounded a call for original scientific studies to "prove the lesion." In 1906 the AOA voted to establish and partially endow a separate institution to serve the dual functions of conducting basic research and teaching advanced courses to D.O.'s already in the field. Opposition to this plan was soon voiced by the colleges, several of which were already offering their own graduate-level classes and felt that the creation of a national center for this purpose would only lure away their students and fees. After three years of wrangling with the schools, the AOA agreed to drop the idea of a teaching role from their proposal, at which point contributions began to be solicited in earnest. In 1913 sufficient funds were raised to purchase and equip a small building in Chicago which became known as the A. T. Still Research Institute.[27]

The first director was John Deason (1874-1946), an American School of Osteopathy alumnus with an M.S. degree from Valparaiso University who had also taken a postgraduate course at the University of Chicago.[28] Several of his experiments and those of his associates centered on producing artificial "bony lesions" upon animal subjects and determining what effect, if any, they would have on certain physiological functions. For the purpose of their research a *bony lesion* was defined as a slight dislocation or subluxation of a vertebra in relation to its adjoining segments. This was induced by manual adjustment of the subject under anesthesia and was verified immediately following and on regular intervals thereafter through digital palpation. Though in the first published compilation of their work they recorded significant changes in carbohydrate metabolism, peristalsis, blood pressure, bile flow, and renal output following these lesions, their evidence establishing causal relationships was less than compelling.[29]

In 1917 a West Coast branch of the institute, headed by Louisa Burns (1868-1958), a 1903 graduate of the Pacific College who later obtained an M.S. degree from the Borden Institute of Indiana, was established outside of Los Angeles.[30] When Deason left basic research for private practice during the first World War, Burns emerged as the profession's only full-time investigator. Her experiments were similar to those that had been carried out by the Chicago group, with some modifications. In her long career, Burns wrote several books and dozens of articles in which she claimed that a variety of functional and organic disturbances of the eyes, heart, lungs, kidneys, stomach, and other viscera were directly attributable to artificially produced lesions that when corrected would allow for a reversal of these other problems.[31] Although many of her D.O. contemporaries were convinced that these studies demonstrated the soundness of their system, knowledgeable critics accurately pointed out that she consistently failed to provide adequate controls and that her conclusions did not generally follow from the data presented.[32] Consequently, as no other basic osteopathic research was being carried out in this era, not even at the colleges, fundamental questions concerning the etiology and role of the lesion in disease remained unsatisfactorily answered.

## The Code of Ethics

In the early days of the movement, rarely did one osteopath locate his practice near that of another, except in the major cities. However, as the number of new D.O.'s increased, it became common for two or more to serve a relatively small town. In such communities, particularly where osteopaths and M.D.'s competed for a limited health dollar, price wars and instances of character assassination took place. These occurrences made osteopathy appear as something other than a lofty calling—an impression furthered by those D.O.'s who engaged in indiscriminate advertising.[33]

In 1904 the AOA adopted a formal code of ethics establishing guidelines for proper professional conduct. This document, based heavily upon the code of the American Medical Association, emphasized cooperation rather than competition. To eliminate price wars, all D.O.'s in a given geographical area were encouraged to formulate definite rules governing "the minimum pecuniary acknowledgement from their patients."[34] This concept was not unheard of within the ranks. Members of the Washington State Osteopathic Association had agreed two years earlier to abide by a uniform fee schedule, charging no less than $2.00 for single office visits, $2.50 for single house calls, and $3.00 for single night visits. Chronic cases were billed $25.00 for the first month, $20.00 for the second, and $15.00 for each subsequent one. Ministers and schoolteachers received special reduced rates, while the poor were to be treated for free.[35] With the AOA now behind this type of arrangement and the Washington plan working to the participants' satisfaction, several other divisional and local societies originated their own schedules.

The code of ethics also prohibited D.O.'s from pirating one another's clients, declaring,

> The physician, in his intercourse with a patient under the care of another physician, should observe the strictest caution and reserve, should give no disingenuous hints relative to the nature and treatment of the patient's disorder, nor should his conduct directly or indirectly tend to diminish the trust reposed in the attending physician. . . . A physician ought not to take care of or treat a patient who has recently been under the care of another osteopathic physician, in the same illness, except in the case of a sudden emergency, or in consultation with the physician previously in attendance or when that physician has relinquished the case or has been dismissed in due form.[36]

Significantly, the code was silent on whether this last courtesy was to be extended to the M.D.'s.

Unethical advertising was denounced in this document as well, and later the AOA published a list of what it found to be the most offensive practices. This included buying newspaper space, publishing field literature that contained a "percentage of cures," and issuing statements the truth of which was open to legal question.[37] The association did not frown on all advertising, however. One type of promotion which was looked upon with great favor was the lay-oriented osteopathic health journal, such as the one established by Henry Stanhope Bunting (1869-1948). Working as a reporter for a Chicago newspaper, Bunting was sent off to Kirksville in the mid-1890s to write a story on Still and his movement. Impressed with what he found, he soon returned to enroll. After graduating in 1900, he settled again in Chicago, where he started a practice and took night classes at a medical college to further his education. In 1901 the busy Dr. Bunting introduced two continuing monthly publications: the *Osteopathic Physician* for the practitioner only, dedicated to voicing all sides of every professional controversy; and *Osteopathic Health,* which was aimed exclusively at the general public. Compared to previous lay literature, the *O.H.,* as it was commonly called, contained little in the hard-sell vein. Instead, there were broad discussions of the philosophy, principles, and practice of osteopathy. Bunting, who maintained an avid interest in advertising theory and wrote a textbook on the subject, believed that the most effective means of getting the attention of people was via the underplayed message.[38] Needless to say, this meant a more dignified approach. A D.O. in the field could send in a list of names and addresses of actual or potential patients, and for a standard fee Bunting would send those so-designated a one-year subscription to *O.H.,* each issue of which would contain a professional card of the practitioner paying for the service. As this system became popular, the AOA in 1914 decided to publish its own lay vehicle, the *Osteopathic Magazine,* which innovatively included nonhealth-related articles. With each of these and other ventures demonstrating their value in generating new business, the desire for and use of more questionable methods greatly diminished.

For those members of the AOA who were unwilling to abide voluntarily by the provisions of the code of ethics, disciplinary action became necessary. Every year the Board of Trustees investigated alleged violations, suspending or expelling those found guilty from its ranks. Not all osteopaths, however, sought membership in the association. In 1918 only 51 percent of some 6,000 listed D.O.'s belonged. In 1930, 57 percent of approximately 7,600 practitioners were in the fold.[39] Thus for several decades almost one-half the total number of D.O.'s were outside the influence or control of the AOA. This gap was filled to some extent by the state osteopathic or medical boards of registration and examination, which had the power to revoke licenses for a variety of reasons coming under the heading of unprofessional conduct. Therefore, although instances of disreputable behavior would continue to be a problem for the movement, organized osteopathy had established the basic institutional mechanisms for dealing with it.

### Impostors and Imitators

By the turn of the century correspondence schools were springing up around the country, particularly where there were no osteopathic practice laws yet in force. In Ohio, for example, a man claiming to be an M.D. as well as a D.O. advertised a teach-yourself-at-home textbook and a handsome diploma, both of which could be purchased for only twenty-five dollars. In New York, where the cost of living was considerably higher, a Norwegian ex-sailor announced a similar service for one hundred dollars.[40] The number of bogus osteopaths thereby produced can only be guessed at; nevertheless, their impact was undeniable. S. C. Matthews, D.O. of Wilkes-Barre, Pennsylvania, complained, "There are towns within my knowledge where disreputable and bungling methods of the unauthorized and uneducated practitioner have so injured the name of our science, that a legitimate osteopath would have the utmost difficulty in establishing himself. At best, it would be a struggle of many weary months."[41]

Since the correspondence schools depended upon newspapers and magazines to attract their "students," the Committee on Education, to whom the AOA Board of Trustees assigned the task of closing them down, decided they would first focus their efforts on the periodicals themselves. The committee reasoned that if publishers were made aware of the absurdity of these charlatans' claims, they would be obligated to refuse to carry their messages. It sent a standard letter: "Would you accept the advertisement of an institution which offered to fit persons for the practice of medicine by a correspondence course of study? Yet it is just as impossible to fit a person by mail for the practice of osteopathy."[42] So that publishers could better appreciate this, the committee attached to their plea a description of the minimum requirements a college needed to obtain AOA approval, plus an abstract of existing statutes. Most of those so contacted wrote back that they would henceforth reject such ads, and by 1907 the committee reported to the Board of Trustees that there remained only one magazine of any sizable circulation that refused to honor their request.[43] Though the selling of mail-order diplomas did not end as a result of the committee's actions, it ceased to be a critical concern of the profession, especially as osteopathic legislation grew more widespread and unearned degrees became worthless as a basis for licensure.

Quite a different problem, however, was presented by those individuals practicing what appeared to many to be osteopathy under a different name. The most numerous were the exponents of chiropractic, founded by Daniel David Palmer (1845-1913). According to Palmer the principles of this system were fashioned by him in 1895, while he was making a living as a magnetic healer in Davenport, Iowa. A janitor who worked in the building where he kept an office told him that he had gone deaf seventeen years earlier after something "gave way" in his back. Reasoning that a displaced vertebra was responsible, Palmer manipulated the spinal segment into its proper position, and the janitor announced that his hearing had returned. Based on this and subsequent cases so treated, Palmer declared that 95 percent of all disease was due to subluxated vertebrae.[44]

In 1898 Palmer began to teach his methods. At first he found few followers, training a total of only fifteen students through 1902, but from then on business started to pick up. However, Daniel David's personal good fortune declined. In 1906 he was convicted of practicing medicine without a license and was sentenced to spend six months in jail. During his incarceration, his school was taken over by his son, Bartlett Joshua Palmer (1881-1961), better known as B.J. When D.D. was released, B.J. squeezed him out of the college, whereupon D.D. tried without success to operate schools elsewhere. Returning to private practice, the elder Palmer wrote a massive textbook, a large portion of which was devoted to a diatribe against his son. Bitter feelings between the two remained strong. At a founder's day parade held in Davenport in August of 1913, the uninvited D.D., marching on foot, was struck from behind by an auto driven by B.J.; D.D. died a few months later, allegedly as a result of his injuries.[45]

Under the younger Palmer the school continued to grow, securing many matriculants by sensational advertising—a practice B.J. encouraged his followers to emulate. By 1916 there reportedly were some fourteen hundred students in attendance, taking one year's training leading to a doctorate in chiropractic, or D.C., degree. For those who could not appear in person, a correspondence course was instituted. As the Davenport college flourished, dozens of other chiropractic schools, the great majority of them engaged in the selling of diplomas, were established across the country.[46]

Many early chiropractors were arrested on the charge of practicing osteopathy without a license. Unlike those with fake D.O. diplomas, however, chiropractors claimed that they were not pretending to be osteopaths and were therefore innocent of any offense. In court they cited a number of differences between the two systems. The D.O.'s, they pointed out, commonly adjusted several vertebrae to treat a given disorder; they invariably adjusted but one. The technique also varied. Osteopathic manipulations were based on the lever principle, namely, the application of pressure on one part of the body to overcome resistance in motion elsewhere. This meant twisting the patient's torso in certain directions while maintaining a steady hold upon the point in structure to be influenced.

The most common chiropractic procedure of the era had the client lying prone with little, if any support below the spine. The operator would then place both hands directly over the subluxated segment and administer a quick thrust downward with all possible force. When D.O.'s were called to the stand, they would often testify that this method was crude and dangrous and would not be employed in osteopathic practice. Ironically, such statements worked to the chiropractors' advantage, since they indicated to juries that there were indeed divergences in approach. With respect to the element of danger, the defendants were only too glad to present patients who had been so treated, attesting to the safety of such maneuvers. To further cement their position, some chiropractors cleverly managed to obtain and circulate signed letters by officials of recognized D.O.-granting schools stating that a course in chiropractic was not the same as one in osteopathy. As a result of these tactics, they generally won acquittal.[47]

Since the courts were beginning to establish the chiropractors' right to engage in their livelihood outside the jurisdiction of either the medical or osteopathic licensure acts, several legislatures realized that unless they passed laws recognizing the group, their states would be inundated with diploma mill graduates. In 1913, despite the vigorous lobbying of M.D.'s and D.O.'s alike, Kansas and Arkansas became the first to enact chiropractic bills. Each required an eighteen-month course of personal instruction at a duly chartered college for licensure. By 1922 twenty other states had similar statutes.[48] At this time the number of D.C.'s legally and illegally in practice probably exceeded the number of legitimate osteopaths in the country. Thus, while the D.O.'s, through the AOA, had made considerable progress in obtaining some professional recognition insofar as certain measures of organization, autonomy, socioeconomic status, and education were concerned, they nevertheless could not prevent the rise of others who were capitalizing upon the therapeutic modality that was the central feature of their own system.

# CHAPTER FIVE

# *Expanding the Scope*

The most controversial issue the D.O.'s wrestled with throughout the first three decades of the twentieth century was their scope of practice, particularly in regard to the range of therapeutic modalities they should utilize and the type of diseases and conditions they should treat. Vying for the support of the majority of practitioners were two distinct groups. One was composed of the self-proclaimed "lesion osteopaths." In their view, Still's system consisted of structural diagnosis and manipulative therapy. They felt that the only thing necessary to do for the patients they saw was find the alleged lesion along the spine or elsewhere and proceed to adjust it. This, after all, was the same approach that Still successfully employed to permit the crippled to throw away their crutches and other chronically ill individuals to lead a more normal life. Opposing this faction were the so-called "broad osteopaths." While these D.O.'s strongly believed in the efficacy of manipulation per se, they were not willing to limit themselves, envisioning the osteopath's role as that of a complete physician able to deal with any case, using whatever means to best help the patient.

## *Surgery and Obstetrics*

The first open debate between the proponents of lesion and broad osteopathy arose over the questions of whether or not the D.O. should receive an education in and practice surgery and obstetrics. Lesion osteopaths argued against their inclusion, principally on the grounds that the D.O. could not be expected to do two or more different tasks as well as he could do one. Why scatter one's energies and attention to other disciplines, no matter how intrinsically worthwhile? If patients were in need of a surgeon or an accoucheur, they could easily be referred to an M.D. specialist. The broad osteopath saw this reasoning as short sighted; if osteopathy was to rank with allopathy, homeopathy, and eclecticism, it was imperative that it provide the same range of services to its clients as they did.

Since the American School of Osteopathy's curriculum did not at first encompass any training in surgery or obstetrics, many early lesionists assumed that their position was in conformity with Still's. However, available evidence strongly suggests that he originally wanted to add these subjects, and once they were integrated in 1897 he gave them his full support.[1] In 1901 he wrote that his students were to be taught all operative surgery commonly performed in rural areas and were to become knowledgeable in the handling of obstetrical cases. "In short," he declared, "our school is prepared and intended to qualify its graduates when called in counsel or to lead that they might have the necessary information at that time so they will not be handicapped or embarrassed."[2]

With the American School of Osteopathy in the lead, the other colleges followed suit. At the time Booth took his survey, all the institutions he visited were conducting classes in obstetrics/gynecology and surgery. When the length of the curriculum was increased, so too were the listed catalog hours devoted to these courses. For the 1908-9 academic year, the Kirksville, Chicago, Philadelphia, and Los Angeles colleges offered a combined average of 293 hours of instruction. By 1918-19, this figure had risen to 802.[4] As this trend became clear, the lesionists gradually, if somewhat reluctantly, came to accept these subjects as legitimate features of osteopathic practice.

Before 1920 comparatively few D.O.'s performed surgery other than setting fractures and closing minor wounds. Poor opportunities for postgraduate education combined with restrictive state licensing laws did not make this field particularly attractive. Significantly, D.O. students who expressed a desire to become surgeons were actually encouraged by their teachers to obtain a valid M.D. degree once they graduated so that they could receive the depth of instruction required and not be legally circumscribed.[5] Obstetrics also constituted a relatively small fraction of the typical osteopath's workload. In 1917 one D.O. took a survey of his colleagues, finding that while 52 percent of those sampled were accepting obstetrical cases, the average practitioner who did handled fewer than five deliveries each year.[6]

A few osteopaths in this era came to specialize in one of the two disciplines, with most of them employing manipulative therapy in their practice, believing that this modality gave them a decided advantage over their M.D. counterparts. In obstetrics, strictly osteopathic procedures were thought to shorten the hours of labor, lessen accompanying pain, prevent mastitis, and secure a more rapid convalescence of the patient.[7] In 1912 Lillian Whiting, D.O. of Los Angeles, published data showing that of ninety-nine primiparae cases who received one to seven months of manipulative treatment prior to birth, the average duration of labor was nine hours and fifty-four minutes, compared to twenty-one hours and six minutes for twenty-four untreated clients, with similar differences noted in multiparae deliveries.[8]

In surgery, Harry L. Collins, D.O., M.D., of the Chicago College claimed

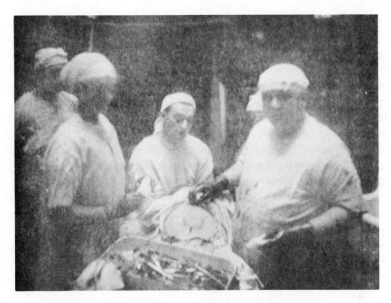

*Rare photo of early osteopathic surgery in progress.*
*The operator at the right is Dr. George Still. (1911)*

that four distinct benefits were to be derived from the osteopathic approach: first, fewer patients needed operations; second, when surgery was indicated the work involved was less extensive than expected of similar cases that had not received previous osteopathic care; third, a D.O. surgeon thoroughly grounded in osteopathic principles was less apt to sacrifice tissues needlessly; and fourth, the postoperative course of the patient ran smoother and encountered fewer complications.[9] Of these assertions, the last was given special emphasis. About 1911 the founder's grandnephew, George A. Still, D.O., M.D. (1882-1922), who had earned his medical diploma and a master's degree in surgery from Northwestern University, began administering manipulative therapy to his clients after they had undergone operations on the theory that this treatment would prevent blood stasis and speed lymphatic absorption, thereby aiding the body's natural defenses against infection. Soon after this program started, a dramatic decline in the rate of surgical pneumonia was recorded. Indeed, Still was so satisfied with these results that he decided to foreswear the common practice of giving strychnine after surgery as a means of stimulating the heart. This seemed only to increase the overall benefits. He told his colleagues, "In our post-operative cases, study the charts and you will see that they do not have the acutely violent cases that usually occur under other treatment. . . . Instead of having a temperature of 105, pulse 165, respiration 70 . . . they are more apt to run a temperature of 102, pulse 120, respiration 35 to 40."[10]

At the same time osteopathic surgeons were broadening the possible applications of manipulative therapy, they were also pointing out when such treatment was contraindicated. In 1904 Frank P. Young, D.O., M.D., then at the American School, wrote a textbook entitled *Surgery from an Osteopathic Standpoint* in which he cautioned against manipulation in ankylosis, dermatitis, hernia, skin ulcers, glanders, cysts, osteomyelitis, scurvy, gangrene, and septicemia. In succeeding years others expanded the list. S. L. Taylor, D.O., M.D., president and surgeon-in-chief at the Des Moines College, observed that five common disorders that osteopaths were treating manipulatively — inflamed tonsils, hemorrhoids, fibroid tumors, gallstones, and appendicitis — were often more successfully handled by the scalpel. James Littlejohn of Chicago argued that in gynecological cases the presence of pustulant inflammatory processes, new growths, displacements, congenital defects, and traumatism signalled surgical and not manipulative intervention, while George A. Still chastised those D.O.'s who adjusted the spine in Pott's disease.[11] As a result of these warnings, D.O.'s became more cognizant of some of the limitations and possible hazards of the founder's methods.

### The Adjuncts Controversy

With the addition of surgery and obstetrics to the curriculum, Still believed his system was complete. His graduates could deal with a wide range of ailments and conditions utilizing all the modalities he felt essential to general practice. The broad osteopaths, however, were not satisfied, looking with favor upon drugless tools such as hydrotherapy, suggestive therapeutics, and electrotherapy, which seemed of value in certain cases. To Still and the lesionists, the employment of these "adjuncts" constituted heresy. In 1902 Still made his feelings known in "Our Platform," an unsigned manifesto consisting of nine campaign planks and offered as the official point of view of the profession. "The fundamental principles of osteopathy," Still declared, "are different from those of any other system and the cause of disease is considered from one standpoint, viz: disease is the result of anatomical abnormalities followed by physiological discord. To cure disease the abnormal parts must be adjusted to the normal, therefore other methods that are entirely different in principle have no place in the osteopathic system."[12]

Responding to this platform, though not to Still personally, was Dain Tasker, D.O. (1872-1964), a graduate of the Pacific College who at the time was completing a book on osteopathic principles which became a standard text in the schools throughout the next thirty years. Of the founder's view of the etiology of disease, Tasker wrote, "This may be the sum of some peoples' osteopathy, but it is not mine. I would really like to know how many men of five years active practice are willing to balance themselves on this two inch strip of a plank. . . . I doubt whether a man who is satisfied with it could be convinced by any line of reasoning whatsoever that life in its manifold phenomena has any other side than the mechanical . . . . FUNCTION DOES AFFECT STRUCTURE JUST AS DECIDEDLY AS STRUCTURE AFFECTS FUNCTION." Turning his attention to adjuncts, Tasker was also direct. "There is no reason," he noted, "why each member of our profession should not feel free to develop and fit himself to aid humanity by the use of sunlight, X-radiance, hydrotherapy or any other method which appeals to his best judgment. . . . In order to be truly scientific we must love truth better than we love our preconceived ideas of what truth is."[13]

The following year, at the 1903 AOA convention in Cleveland, this controversy came to a head when Dr. William Smith took the floor and began ridiculing his colleagues for some of the modalities they were using. "I gave up medical practice and why?" he rhetorically asked. "Because I thought I got something better. . . . And so today when I look around me and I see so many adjuncts to osteopathy, when I find this man using the colon tube, and the other man using the vibrator to treat the eyes, and a third using electric massage to fix up a patient's back, another man with a static apparatus to restore manhood . . . and another with something to grow hair on bald heads, I ask you where in the name of common sense is osteopathy in all that?" Smith was immediately seconded by Herbert Bernard, D.O. of Detroit, who observed, "At this stage of osteopathic history, when there is so little known and so much to learn, is it not foolish to tie to the osteopathic kite a tail made up of electrotherapeutics, hydrotherapy, with a few other adjunct knots tied in it? People in looking at it from a distance might mistake the tail for the kite. They, the people, are very likely to call osteopathy anything else but what it is anyway. Is it, can it be possible, that some of us are helping them to do this?"[14]

The defenders of the adjuncts in turn claimed that their opponents gave manipulation too much credit. C. W. Young, D.O., a graduate of the Northern School, noted, "Dr. Smith spoke of the use of the colon tube. I have interviewed a number of Kirksville graduates in Minneapolis and St. Paul and I have listened to their talk pertaining to this matter but I have never yet learned any purely manipulative method which will invariably move feces in the colon. And if it was one who was near and dear to me above everything else that Dr. Smith was called to treat, and some hot water and the colon tube would save that life, and he refrained from using them in order to stand by osteopathy, I would not think of him as being much less than a murderer." Responding to Young's harsh attack on Smith, C. M. T. Hulett caustically implied that the former's education left something to be desired: "Now then, Dr. Young never studied under Dr. Still. He got his osteopathy second hand. It may be just as good, but when he asserts that osteopathy as taught by Dr. Still is deficient, he must prove that Dr. Still and those men [he instructed] failed, not that he failed in order to substantiate his position."[15]

Though this debate was largely fought between American School of Osteopathy graduates and the alumni of other schools, many of which had already integrated one or more adjuncts into their curriculum, the Kirksville group was by no means of one mind. Carl P. McConnell, the author of a major manual on osteopathic practice in which he attempted to reconcile Still's ideas with that of the distinguished physician William Osler, had declared on a previous occasion:

> While I am perfectly willing to concede the major part of what our therapeutics should be to manipulation, I am by no means willing to assert that every disease or ailment of the body means "readjustment" of certain tissues, in order to restore health. I have heard one or two argue that it makes no difference whatever one uses as food provided his vertebrae, ribs, etc. are in correct position. It would be quite laughable, if it were not so serious to hear such narrow-mindedness. If their proposition were true, medical knowledge prior to the discovery of osteopathy amounted to naught. They do not seem to realize that it was through medical knowledge already existing that osteopathy was developed. It is just such people as this that harm us more before the medical world and public more than anything else. They will bring up their "manipulative argument" when they do not have the first conception of hygiene, preventative medicine, etc.[16]

With opinion sharply divided, no consensus was obtained on the adjuncts issue at the convention. Given a lack of policy directive, it was left to individual schools and practitioners to decide their own course. In the ensuing years the lesionists were encouraged by the discarding or avoidance of some adjuncts by most of their colleagues; however, sentiment had clearly shifted towards the position of the broad osteopath on others.[17] Indeed, certain agencies became so acceptable—hydrotherapy, corrective exercise, diet and food chemistry, and mental therapeutics—that in 1912 the *JAOA* introduced new regular monthly columns on each. Although these and other drugless modalities came to occupy only a minor place in the college curricula and in patient management, their integration was nevertheless important since it marked the first significant divergence by the majority of the profession from the original doctrines and charismatic authority of Still.

### Chemical and Biological Agents

While the questions of whether surgery, obstetrics, and the so-called adjuncts should become part of the osteopathic system were decided relatively quickly, the issue of chemicals, vaccines, serums, and endocrines followed a less easy path to resolution. Despite the fact that the same principles put forward in the adjuncts controversy were relevant here, namely the freedom of the practitioner to choose any modality thought helpful in the management of a given disorder and the right of the schools to teach what they desired, the symbolic meaning of chemical and biological weapons to the pioneers of the movement made this a lengthier and more painful matter to settle.

The last third of the nineteenth century was marked by several momentous changes in the practice of orthodox medicine. With each passing year an increasing percentage of regulars came to rely on a smaller number of drugs in less heroic doses for those conditions in which they seemed indicated.[18] Though as late as 1899 the *Merck Manual of Therapeutics* listed sixty-eight different treatments for diabetes mellitus—including arsenic "for thin subjects," codeine ("a most effective remedy sometimes requires to be pushed to the extent of 10 grains per day"), iron ("most useful with morphine"), and belladonna "full doses"—the great majority of American M.D.'s were rejecting this empirical approach.[19] Medical thought was also transformed by the emerging fields of bacteriology and immunology and the work of such scientists as Pasteur, Koch, Behring, and Erlich, who shifted the focus of practice from eliminating the symptoms of infection to destroying or rendering inert pathogenic microorganisms and their byproducts. This was made possible largely through vaccines, which allowed the patient to manufacture his own antibodies, and serums, which already contained the specific antibodies of another human or animal.[20] By 1900 effective prophylactic and therapeutic agencies for rabies (1885), diphtheria (1891), tetanus (1891), cholera (1892), plague (1897), and typhoid fever (1898) had been developed.

Still, for his part, was unimpressed by these advances, believing that the chemical and biological tools employed by the M.D.'s were often toxic to the body, as well as being vile and disgusting.[21] Furthermore, the regulars were ignoring the structural basis of disease. One might conceivably eliminate symptoms through such modalities, but not the underlying cause, namely, lesions. Finally, whatever the alleged usefulness of these weapons, osteopathy was always equal to the task. Still claimed, for example, that he could prevent the chills and fever of malaria without quinine by periodically adjusting the lumbar vertebrae; disperse the fluid in dropsy without digitalis by treating the eleventh and twelfth ribs; and reduce the swelling of a gouty big toe without colchicine by manipulating the foot. As for the diphtheria antitoxin, his son Charles had proven in Red Wing, Minnesota, that a D.O. could get spectacular results without it.[22] The only orthodox medicinal agencies Still did sanction were anesthetics and antiseptics in surgical and obstetrical practice, and antidotes in poisoning cases.[23]

Those who were in favor of adopting a wider variety of drugs, including vaccines, serums, and endocrines, seemed at first to be mainly D.O.'s who also held a medical degree. Their additional training and experience had convinced them that some of these tools had proven their worth and that there was no valid reason for not using them in total patient management. If a client was suffering from gout, it made sense to them to both manipulate and administer colchicine. Similarly, in malaria, why not adjust the spine and give quinine together? In this fashion, the client would receive the best of both systems.

Still did not think much of this view. In 1903 he rhetorically asked,

> What will become of the M.D. D.O.? He ought to be put in a class by himself and no doubt will be if he attempts to practice osteopathy and medicine combined. . . . Medicine and osteopathy as therapeutical agencies have nothing in common either theoretically or practically, and only an inconsistent physician will attempt to practice both. Osteopathy does not need to be bolstered up by the use of any therapeutical knowledge to be learned at any medical school. Each state association should adopt such rules as will require the resignation of all two-faced practitioners and prevent them from being taken in hereafter. Osteopaths cannot afford to compromise their position in regard to drug medication and should bar from their association all mixers and their ilk, who honor neither the profession of osteopathy nor medicine.[24]

In 1905 such an event took place when the Illinois Osteopathic Association asked one of its members, W. A. Hinckle, D.O., M.D., to resign. In an eloquent reply he wrote:

> Being a physician and not a sectarian practitioner I am heir to and privileged to make use of any and all therapeutic measures which the accumulated knowledge of centuries has shown to be of value, or which future learning may place within my reach regardless of its source or character. . . . Every physician must decide from his own experience and from the experience of others as to the relative value of the curative measures at hand and on the breadth of his learning, the accuracy of his judgment and his freedom to choose will decide his stature as a physician. This freedom your president informs me is neither desired nor permitted in your society, I am given to understand that you prefer to share fellowship only with those who choose limitations rather than freedom. As membership in your society can therefore be purchased only at the price of intellectual liberty, I hereby present you with my resignation preferring rather the glorious isolation of unfettered thoughts and activities than the company of those who are slaves to creed and dogma.[25]

In spite of this organizational push to impose therapeutic purity by the Illinois association as well as other state societies, more D.O.'s were beginning to question the wisdom of rejecting all chemicals and biologicals. With the statistics gathered from repeated clinical trials demonstrating the efficacy of these proscribed agencies, the rationale upon which an osteopath could shun them became far more difficult to defend.[26] Some practitioners were forced to reconsider when they themselves encountered failure in treating patients with manipulation. In 1908 Frank I. Furry, D.O., M.D., and then vice-president of the AOA, told his colleagues of his own dilemma in caring for his daughter, who had contracted diphtheria:

I had kept myself reasonably well posted on the serum therapy . . . and was opposed to the use of antitoxin. I chose osteopathy straight and we fought it out on that line and lost. No internal medication was used, excepting a hypodermic injection of strychnine to support the heart during the intubation process at the last. . . . The specialist who performed the intubation . . . called me a criminal in the presence of my dying child because I had not used antitoxin (which he claimed to be an absolute specific) and since thinking the matter over I do not know but that every member of our profession is a criminal just to the extent that he has failed to assist in the solution of this awful problem.[27]

From the beginning of the century all of the colleges were exposing their students to information about biologicals and chemicals through their courses in toxicology, surgery, obstetrics, and practice, since for the most part they were using the same textbooks employed in orthodox institutions. Though many teachers ignored or attacked the sections of such works dealing with the supposed benefits of these agencies except for anesthetics, antiseptics, and antidotes, other institutions appeared less dogmatic. In 1906 Charles C. Teall, D.O., who had succeeded Booth as the AOA inspector of schools, complained that too many medical notations were finding their way into the lectures. At Chicago, "'Broad Osteopathy' a science embracing everything was talked by the president of the senior class." In Boston, "elaborate detail in antiseptic, medicated douches, lotions, etc. is given, while the osteopathic part is taken for granted with 'of course find the lesion and remove.'" At Los Angeles, "certain formulas were on the board and copied by the students which will land them in jail, or at least give them trouble if used in most any state of the union for it was strict medical practice."[28]

In defending their schools, a number of faculty members and administrators argued that there should be some classroom discussion of chemicals and biologicals so that students could intelligently decide the merits of their use for themselves. Furthermore, it appeared to them that even more instruction in these modalities would have to be given, whether they liked it or not, if their graduates were to secure greater legal privileges insofar as surgery and obstetrics were concerned. In Illinois, for example, the medical act allowed for the granting of two types of licenses, one for a physician and surgeon and the other for a drugless practitioner. To be eligible for the first, candidates had to have graduated from schools approved by the state board of health, which required the inclusion of a complete course in *materia medica*. Supporters of the Chicago school tried to change the law, but repeatedly failed. Consequently, in 1909 the college attempted to comply by adding "osteopathic *materia medica*" to the curriculum. It then applied for recognition but was turned down on the grounds that the subject was not being adequately taught. The Littlejohns sued the board but eventually lost their case, whereupon ownership of the institution was transferred and the course was dropped.[29]

A similar situation occurred in California with a different outcome. Since 1906 D.O.'s had been able to secure full physicians and surgeons certification if they passed the same test required of M.D.'s. However, in 1913 the law was amended to stipulate that anyone wishing to take the examination had to be a graduate of a college giving a minimum number of hours in specified subjects, including pharmacology. The Los Angeles school therefore made the necessary changes and thus became approved by the composite California Medical Board.[30]

While the Chicago and Los Angeles colleges represented extreme cases, the other schools were also expanding their curricula. Both Philadelphia and Boston offered optional courses on *materia medica* which did not appear in their annual catalogs.[31] Des Moines introduced a series of lectures in "Comparative Therapeutics" which it defended on the grounds that "in this way the osteopath will be better able to explain the practice of osteopathy to the minds of a public used to drugs."[32] Even Kirksville, after the founder retired from active control, began moving into previously prohibited areas. In 1911 its catalog description of the course in bacteriology noted, "vaccines, antitoxins and serum therapy with the values and ill effects resulting from the careless or improper use of each in practice are specifically and logically taught."[33]

These straightforward and roundabout efforts at integrating chemicals and biologicals into the curricula were naturally opposed by the lesionists, a number of whom held important positions within the AOA hierarchy. At first they tried to cajole the colleges into withdrawing these subjects, but when this seemed a waste of time they decided to follow a more drastic course. At the 1915 convention in Philadelphia the Board of Trustees ruled that after 1916 "engaging in the teaching of drug therapeutics by any member of this association shall be cause for depriving of membership in this organization; and that participation in such training by any college shall be cause for refusal by the Association for recognition of such colleges as a cooperating institution."[34] Several months later the board supported the successful lobbying efforts of a group of Oregon D.O.'s who secured an amendment to their existing law which stated, "No school of osteopathy whose curriculum includes a course of materia medica, pharmacology or prescription writing is to be considered for the purpose of this act to be a regularly conducted school of osteopathy."[35]

Protest within the ranks both nationally and in Oregon soon followed. Listing a number of orthodox remedies for his colleagues to consider, Henry

Bunting, publisher of the *Osteopathic Physician,* asked for a definition of *materia medica.*

> If you had an elderly patient whose body was eaten out with malignant cancer, dying by inches, would you yield to her entreaties and give her morphine? If you had a son who was a cretin would you give him thyroid extract? If your child had diphtheria would you use antitoxin? If bitten by a mad dog would you yourself take the Pasteur treatment? If you had a patient bleeding to death would you blanche the wound with adrenalin? . . . Would you use pumpkin seed to expel a tapeworm? Would you give an anemic organized iron? If you had a syphilitic patient would you use mercury or salvarsan or anything else now used to help that condition? . . . If you had a patient whose heart beat about 160 and you weren't sure the pulse was strong enough to count would you ever wonder if digitalis might not be a help in that one case?[36]

With Bunting for the first time publicly declaring himself to be in favor of teaching the use of biological and chemical agencies in the colleges, other D.O.'s who previously had been silent on this issue voiced their support. They were joined by those who, while not in favor of a separate course in *materia medica,* were nonetheless opposed to the board's ruling and the Oregon law on the grounds that neither the AOA nor the state legislatures had any business interfering with the colleges' right to determine their educational policy.[37]

With opinion steadily mounting in a direction favoring the teaching of *materia medica,* the founder, now eighty-seven years old, made an open appeal to his followers just before the start of the 1915 convention in Portland, where this matter was sure to be raised. Still warned, "There is an alarm at the door of all osteopathic schools. The enemy has broken through the picket. Shall we permit the osteopathic profession to be enslaved to the medical truth? As the father of osteopathy, I am making an international call for all Simon-pure D.O.'s who are willing to go on the fighting line without being drafted into service."[38] Still's plea was unsuccessful. Bowing to pressure from its critics, the Board of Trustees revoked the previous year's directive, thus in effect both disavowing itself from the Oregon law and leaving the colleges free to teach what they wanted.[39] Slowly, the profession was coming out from under Still's shadow.

Although this action seemed to signal the dawn of a new era for the movement, a rather extraordinary chain of events occurred soon afterwards which temporarily restored the lesionists to power. In 1918 and 1919 some 650 thousand persons in the United States and approximately 40 million worldwide died as a result of what was known as the swine flu, a particularly lethal strain of influenza virus which had surfaced after several decades of dormancy.[40] No specific vaccine or serum had been developed, nor was there any effective drug therapy that could shorten or minimize the course of the disease. In their treatment of the afflicted, most American physicians proceeded cautiously, isolating the patient, establishing satisfactory hygienic conditions, and carefully regulating fluid intake. Drugs were used only to relieve symptoms, as in the more common forms of influenza. Those relying on Osler's textbook, for example, gave a dose of calomel during the day to open the bowels, ten grains of Dover's powders at night to relieve the aches and pains, aspirin to reduce the fever, and strychnine full doses in cases manifesting great cardiac weakness.[41]

Most D.O.'s, on the other hand, while generally following orthodox procedures with respect to isolation, hygiene, and fluid intake, rejected drugs altogether, substituting manipulative measures in their place. Such therapy directed at the spine and rib cage would, according to its advocates, help normalize visceral functions and specifically build up resistance to and disperse fluid in pneumonia, which was a common sequela.[42] With many D.O.'s in the field at the beginning of the pandemic reporting to their journals on how well they seemed to be doing in comparison to local M.D.'s, a campaign to gather and publish statistics was launched and given wide publicity in the *Osteopathic Physician* and *JAOA*. Between October, 1918, and June, 1919, a total of 2,445 D.O.'s mailed in a summary of their results and a general description of their approach. Of 110,120 influenza cases compiled during this period, there were but 257 deaths listed (a .2 percent mortality). Of 6,258 pneumonia reports, there were only 635 fatalities (a 10.1 percent mortality). These figures were compared to an estimated 12 to 15 percent influenza and 25 percent pneumonia death rate of patients under the care of orthodox physicians.[43] Although the adequacy of their data collection methods and conclusions was laid open to serious question by the M.D.'s, the D.O.'s were convinced that they had documented their therapeutic superiority.[44]

The impact of this experience upon the members of the profession was quite significant, as many of those who had doubted the applicability of manipulative therapy in the management of acute infectious diseases began treating such cases with their hands. Furthermore, as a result of surviving the flu, or knowing someone who had, patients who had previously patronized the osteopath only for joint and muscle disturbances, as well as individuals who had never frequented the office of an osteopath, now decided that they would rely on the D.O. as their family doctor. Manipulative therapy was again on the rise.

With sentiments towards biological and chemical agencies thereby diminishing, those D.O.'s who were behind or supported the 1914 resolution and Oregon amendment reasserted themselves. In 1920 the Board of Trustees and the House of Delegates passed "The Profession's Policy," which attempted to set definite restrictions on the D.O.'s scope of practice. One section of this document embodied a standard college curriculum covering what it called "all the subjects necessary to educate a thoroughly competent general osteopathic practitioner." Neither pharmacology nor *materia medica* was listed. Training in certain types of drugs, including germicides and parasiticides, was to be given, but no mention was made of other chemotherapeutic agents such as digitalis, colchicine, or vaccines, serums, and endocrines. A second section concerning legislation called for a revision of the model bill, incorporating language in each state law to limit licensees to use only those drugs as "taught in the standard college curriculum which means the standard curriculum of the A.O.A." Rather than oppose these new proscriptions, school officials cooperated in their formulation.[45] Apparently the renaissance in the osteopathic fundamentalism had influenced them as it had practitioners in the field.

Nevertheless, once the initial wave of enthusiasm had passed, dissatisfaction with the new policy became evident. The broad osteopaths, ending a discreet period of silence, again took the offensive, blasting away at what they felt was the intellectual vacuousness of the AOA position. However, more practitioners seemed to be upset by the adverse affect the policy had on their efforts to obtain favorable laws. A majority of state legislatures continued to reject attempts to expand the legal scope of osteopathic practice vis-à-vis surgery and obstetrics as well as those drugs the AOA sanctioned. Many representatives simply refused to budge from their long-held view that before they would seriously consider their requests, the D.O.'s would have to demonstrate that they received the same breadth of undergraduate training as did the M.D.'s. This meant teaching the use of all generally recognized preventive and therapeutic measures.[46] Rather than blame the legislators, these D.O.'s turned their wrath on the AOA leadership, arguing that in its stubborn insistence upon a limited instruction in biological and chemical therapy it was biting its nose off to spite its face.

In 1924, due to strong student pressure, administrators of the Chicago College announced that it would once again attempt to meet legislative demands by adding a comprehensive course in *materia medica* to the curriculum. E. S. Comstock, D.O., secretary of the school, declared, "If we have sufficient faith in the osteopathic concept and in osteopathic principles, if they are sufficiently convincing to the logic and intelligence of the average human being, why should we fear the knowledge of drug action, when so often the untoward results outnumber the beneficial effects." The AOA board, however, was unimpressed, voting seventeen to one against such a course in osteopathic colleges, thus causing the Chicago school, threatened with a loss of its accreditation, to back down.[47]

The board's decision in this case helped to fuel the opposition. With increasing numbers of D.O.'s in the field resenting anyone placing a restriction on their scope of practice, and with some of the schools seemingly on the verge of openly defying the provisions of the standard curriculum, the AOA leadership began to realize that a reconsideration of the issue was necessary. In July, 1927, members of the board met with representatives of the Associated Colleges and hammered out a compromise. That fall each school, with the board's blessing, would begin teaching a course called "comparative therapeutics." What this would include was not made explicit; nevertheless, it was thought that the title would satisfy the lawmakers.[48] Initial reaction, however, proved otherwise, with some in government characterizing it as a mere subterfuge.[49]

Frustration within the ranks mounted. Scathing letters from prominent D.O.'s against the amended policy filled the pages of osteopathic publications, while a few state societies formally demanded that the board immediately make the necessary changes.[50] Given this steady bombardment of criticism, the board met with college officials once more in the summer of 1929. This time they agreed to an outline of a course called "supplementary therapeutics," which specifically mandated complete training in the use of biological and chemical agencies. This proposal was then submitted to the AOA House of Delegates, which had the final say. It decided to make sure the legislatures knew what the phrase *supplementary therapeutics* meant by adding *pharmacology* as one of its subheadings.[51] As a few of the more conservative colleges felt that adding pharmacology per se was going too far, the house the next year made its teaching "permissable" rather than "required."[52] Nevertheless, the significance of the 1929 resolution remained undiminished. The official policy of the AOA was now finally and irreversibly in favor of a truly complete and unlimited scope of practice.

# CHAPTER SIX

# *The Push for Higher Standards*

With D.O.'s increasingly duplicating the role and services of M.D.'s the focus of the debate over the relative merits of osteopathy gradually shifted from its underlying philosophical and therapeutical beliefs to an analysis of its educational system. The central question became whether the standards maintained by osteopathic colleges were adequate to ensure the production of qualified physicians and surgeons.

### The Revolution in Medical Education

The issue of standards did not apply solely to osteopathy. At the turn of the century medical education in the United States was noted for its disparities. On one end of the continuum were a relatively small number of prestigious university-affiliated colleges, on the other were the profit-motivated proprietary schools. Despite the gulf between the two types of institutions in terms of staffing, facilities, and equipment, licensing laws made it as easy for the graduates of one type to obtain the right to practice as it did the graduates of the other. Most existing boards of registration and examination either did not have the power to set meaningful standards for the colleges or had declined to do so.[1]

In 1904 the recently reorganized AMA formed a Council on Medical Education to suggest methods of improving academic requirements and to serve as an ongoing agency for advancing the association's policies. In order to determine the actual situation in the colleges, the AMA Board of Trustees the following year authorized the council to undertake a complete on-site survey and rate all 160 M.D.-granting schools. Although the grading was reportedly lenient, only 82 were given Class A, or approved, ranking; 46 were placed on Class B, or probation; and 32 were designated as Class C, or unapproved. While this information was not revealed to the public, it was made available to each state licensing board for its consideration; as a result a number decided they would henceforth refuse to examine graduates of schools not receiving the council's approval. Several colleges were thus motivated to begin making needed improvements and others simply shut their doors. Between 1906 and 1910, the number of M.D.-granting institutions decreased by twenty-nine.[2]

The lay public's first detailed knowledge of the still generally lamentable school conditions came with the publication of Abraham Flexner's *Medical Education in the United States and Canada* (1910), an on-site survey carried out under the auspices of the Carnegie Foundation for the Advancement of Teaching and in cooperation with the AMA council. Though Flexner found some colleges upholding what he considered to be satisfactory standards, these constituted a decided minority. With respect to matriculation, only one of four was insisting upon either a high school diploma or liberal arts college credit as the minimum prerequisite for admission; the remainder were permitting even the barely literate to enroll. Most schools lacked fully equipped research laboratories for the first two years of instruction, and in the third and fourth years too many students were not being given the necessary hospital and dispensary experience to prepare them for practice.[3]

In his report Flexner suggested several reforms. First, he urged that all proprietary schools be closed down. Since the United States then had far more M.D.'s per 100,000 people than the industrialized European nations, it was unlikely that the loss of these institutions and their graduates would lead to any physician shortage. He further recommended that each college worth keeping open become an integral component of a major university, thus ensuring higher academic standards. Finally, he strongly suggested that the financing of medical education be altered. Since tuition fees could only cover a fraction of the expenses necessary to support an adequate program, other sources of income had to be cultivated.[4]

This survey had a considerable impact upon the American consciousness. In the era of muckraking journalism, Flexner's overall findings and vivid descriptions of individual schools made excellent copy and were widely circulated by the nation's press. Now in a position to mobilize public opinion, the various groups committed to change went forward in their efforts to accelerate the progress already being made.[5] In the twenty-five years following the appearance of the Carnegie Foundation study several significant improvements were made along the lines Flexner laid down. First, the number of schools steadily dropped. Commercial and otherwise weak institutions were forced out of business as more state boards accepted the continually updated ratings of the Council on Medical Education.[6] By 1935 there were but sixty-six AMA-accredited colleges, fifty-seven of which were connected with a university.[7]

Higher entrance standards were also set and maintained. In 1918 the council ruled that all incoming students had to have completed two years of college work. As of 1936, 83.3 percent of all matriculants exceeded this minimum, while 48.7 percent enrolled with a baccalaureate degree. The educational program itself was greatly enhanced, this due in large part to the changes in the colleges' fiscal condition. During the 1934-35 and 1935-36 academic years, 55.3 percent of the total income of all medical schools was raised through taxes, public and private general university funds, and philanthropy.[8] With the additional revenue these sources brought, the colleges built more completely outfitted laboratories, hired full-time basic science instructors (mostly Ph.D.'s), and upgraded their hospital and dispensary facilities.

These advances helped spur considerable progress on the postdoctoral level. With the schools' rise in quality, graduate programs ceased being undergraduate repair shops.[9] In 1912 the council conducted its first inspection of hospitals offering internships. From then through the mid-1930s, standards were regularly strengthened as this additional year of training became all but obligatory.[10] In 1927 the council published its first list of approved residencies, and in 1933 the AMA established the organizational machinery to create boards of certification in the various specialties. These changes, along with those on the predoctoral level, would provide the American people with a more uniform corps of highly skilled M.D.'s.

### Osteopathic Evolution

In his grand tour of the nation's medical schools, Flexner decided to include osteopathic colleges on his itinerary. In spite of the differences in approach between D.O.'s and M.D.'s, Flexner believed that the D.O. teaching centers should be surveyed, declaring, "Whatever his notions on the subject of treatment, the osteopath needs to be trained to recognize disease and to differentiate one disease from another quite as carefully as any other medical practitioner. . . . Whether they use drugs or do not use them, whether some use them while others do not does not affect this fundamental question. . . . All physicians summoned to see the sick are confronted with precisely the same crisis: a body out of order. No matter what remedial measures they incline—medical, surgical, manipulative—they must ascertain what is the trouble. There is only one way to do that. The osteopaths admit it when they teach physiology, pathology, chemistry, microscopy."[11]

Having placed the movement for the purpose of his analysis on an equal footing with orthodox medicine, Flexner was quick to emphasize that not one "of the eight osteopathic schools is in a position to give such training as osteopathy demands." The teaching of anatomy, for example, was "fatally defective." Most of the students' time during this course was spent listening to lectures; too few cadavers were available to provide adequate laboratory dissection. This pattern characterized the other basic sciences as well. "A small chemical laboratory is occasionally seen," Flexner noted.

At Philadelphia it happens to be in a dark cellar. At Kirksville, a fair sized room is devoted to pathology and bacteriology; the huge classes are divided into bands of 32, each of which gets a six weeks course following the directions of a rigid syllabus, under a teacher who is himself a student. . . . A professor at the Kansas City school [the Central College] said of his own institution that it had practically no laboratories at all; the Still College at Des Moines has in place of laboratories laboratory signs; the Littlejohn at Chicago, whose catalog avers that the "physician should be imbued with a knowledge of the healing arts in its widest fields, and here is the opportunity" has lately in rebuilding wrecked all its laboratories but that of chemistry without in the least interfering with its usual pedagogic routine.

Clinical instruction fared no better. "The osteopath," he declared, "cannot learn his technique and when it is applicable except through experience with ailing individuals. And these for the most part he begins to see only . . . after receiving his D.O. degree." Bedside training was, in fact, either very limited or nonexistent. Kirksville had the largest hospital, a mere fifty-four beds, while Chicago had twenty, the Pacific College fifteen, Boston ten, and Philadelphia three. Des Moines, Kansas City, and Los Angeles had none at the time of his visit. Outpatient contact was similarly restricted. Each of the colleges operated a pay clinic that was staffed by the faculty and in which student participation seems to have been limited to the care of charity cases.[12]

In characterizing the entire educational program, Flexner wrote:

The eight osteopathic schools now enroll over 1,300 students who pay some $200,000 annually in fees. The instruction furnished for this sum is inexpensive and worthless. Not a single full time teacher is found in any of them. The fees find their way directly into the pockets of the school owners, or into school buildings, and infirmaries that are equally their property. No effort is anywhere made to utilize prosperity as a means of defining an entrance standard or developing the "science." Granting all that its champions claim, osteopathy is still in its incipiency. If sincere its votaries would be engaged in critically building it up. They are doing nothing of the kind.[13]

Angry protests by school officials and other D.O.'s greeted the publication of Flexner's report. Responding to his critique, the AOA Board of Trustees declared, "We have no apologies to offer for our colleges. They have done well, and we take pride in their attainments and in their ambitions and determinations to teach most thoroughly and scientifically all that pertains to disease in all its phases and manifestations. We demand that they be allowed to do this, according to the needs of our profession and not in accord with the wishes of any self-appointed, self-seeking, tyrannical and prejudicial judges."[14] Interestingly, this view was not completely shared by the AOA

Committee on Education. In its annual report for 1910, it substantially agreed with Flexner on the problems of low entrance standards, poor basic science laboratories, lack of sufficient clinical facilities, and an inadequate teaching corps, as its own surveys had noted the same deficiencies, albeit in less caustic language.[15] However, unlike Flexner, who evaluated the schools with an ideal in mind, D.O. inspectors considered themselves pragmatic to the extent that they recognized the limited possibilities for amelioration under existing conditions. Reform, they believed, would have to be slow.

The twenty-five years following the issuance of the Flexner report saw some improvements in college requirements and in the quality of training offered; nevertheless, osteopathic institutions did not keep pace with the changes engineered by the M.D.'s. With respect to preprofessional education, the AOA Board of Trustees in 1920 stipulated that henceforth each school must maintain an entrance standard of no less than a high school diploma or its equivalent to keep its accreditation rating, yet no attempt was immediately made to enforce this provision, and it was not until the early 1930s that all the schools appeared to be fully complying.[16] Those in favor of further stringency in entrance requirements were a decided minority. Los Angeles established a compulsory one year of college qualification in 1920, but this was only in response to a California law mandating it. Most D.O.'s sided with Dr. George Laughlin, who in 1925 observed, "We make a mistake as a profession when we attempt to ape the medical man in matters of requirements."[17] Laughlin, the founder's son-in-law and now head of the Kirksville College, argued that the two years of prior college work was hurting the underprivileged since they could least afford the cost of additional schooling. As many of these disappointed students came from farms and small towns, the standard had the indirect effect of causing a decline in the percentage of recent M.D. graduates deciding to locate in sparsely populated areas. Without this qualification, D.O. schools could meet the needs of the economically disadvantaged student and help alleviate the growing rural physician shortage.[18]

Whatever the merits of Laughlin's views, the main reason militating against a further increase in preprofessional requirements was the economic condition of the colleges themselves. Although all of the schools had emerged as nonprofit institutions, the sources of their funding remained the same. They received no direct tax support, no general university monies, and in comparison with M.D. institutions, little outside philanthropy. In 1932 reportedly 92 percent of the gross receipts of all the colleges were secured from tuition fees alone.[19] Given this form of operation, the schools' very survival depended on their ability to obtain a base line of new matriculants each fall. By setting the preprofessional standard at the M.D.'s level of two years or more, the osteopathic schools would drastically cut their pool of eligible applicants, and their quota of students necessary to meet expenses would very likely not be reached.[20]

During this era a large percentage of the schools' annual tuition income was devoted to establishing more permanent facilities. In 1921 the Los Angeles College moved to a new campus where three large buildings were erected over the next decade. The Kansas City College of Osteopathy and Surgery, founded in 1916, had two homes before finding a suitable location four years later, where it raised five new structures by 1933.[21] The Chicago school left the downtown area for the Hyde Park section of the city in 1918, renovating a large four-story working girls' residence to provide classrooms, laboratory, hospital, and clinic space. The Des Moines College in 1927 relocated from one entire office building to another, while the American School of Osteopathy, whose name was changed to the Kirksville College of Osteopathy and Surgery, added a new facility for laboratories and classrooms along with a second hospital. Only the Philadelphia school, which in 1929 established a new campus costing $1.1 million, was able to finance its plans through private donations.[22]

The educational program of the schools underwent a number of important changes between 1910 and 1935. The colleges added a mandatory fourth year, introduced a graded curriculum, and integrated biological and chemical therapy to the course of study. As a result, in its promotional literature the profession could boast that in terms of subjects presented and time devoted to them, M.D. and D.O. schools were equivalent. Indeed, on paper osteopathic institutions offered students a few hundred more hours of training than the typical orthodox college. However, this was a deceptive figure; although the length of basic science courses in D.O. schools was greatly expanded, the instruction itself continued to be weak.[23] By the early 1930s most preclinical teachers were full time, but few of these D.O.'s possessed a graduate degree in the subjects they taught. Their new buildings provided more adequate facilities, yet the equipment remained meager, and most laboratories were fitted out with the barest of necessities. Money that could have purchased additional, improved apparatus had to be diverted into mortgage payments. Finally, the courses were often not as encompassing as those in allopathic colleges, partly because the preprofessional backgrounds of M.D. and D.O. matriculants differed. Osteopathic curricula, for example, included elementary biology and chemistry, which medical students had mastered before beginning their formal professional education.

Clinical training was also beset by severe difficulties. All of the schools were operating larger hospitals in the mid-thirties than previously; however, most were still quite small. While most M.D. colleges easily surpassed the minimum of 200 beds available for teaching purposes under guidelines set by the AMA council,[24] the Chicago, Des Moines, Kansas City, Kirksville, and Philadelphia schools of osteopathy averaged only sixty-six apiece.[25]

Thus, where a minimum of 2,000 curriculum hours were devoted to bedside and outpatient teaching at most M.D.-granting institutions, an average of approximately seven hundred hours was spent at these five colleges.[26]

The one osteopathic school that was able to provide clinical training approaching that found in orthodox colleges was Los Angeles. This was made possible through its utilization of a 203-bed public hospital, which enabled each student to receive 1,770 hours of inpatient dispensary experience.[27] The establishment of this institution was an unintended by-product of the "standardization of hospitals" plan inaugurated by the American College of Surgeons in 1918 and later pursued by the AMA. Any hospital seeking the approval of these groups was required to prohibit D.O.'s from having admitting or staff privileges. As a result, osteopaths throughout the country who had managed to secure such rights found them abruptly terminated.[28] The county government, due to pressure from the D.O.'s and their supporters, opened a separate public hospital for the use of the Los Angeles School, which was now denied access to the public facility.[29] Unfortunately for the profession, this type of arrangement was not repeated elsewhere.

With clinical experience in the colleges generally limited, it is hardly surprising that postgraduate training was also far from satisfactory. By the middle 1930s there were no more than eighty osteopathic hospitals in the country, of which only one-quarter were offering opportunities for advanced work.[30] In 1932 there were but seventy-five internships, few approaching the standards governing M.D. programs.[31] Formal residencies were even more scarce. Those osteopaths who could not enter one of these had to learn their specialty by attending short courses given at the colleges or by taking a preceptorship with a private practitioner. Clearly, such conditions as well as those on the undergraduate level left much to be desired.

## The Price of Lower Standards

Although osteopathic colleges during most of this period attempted to prepare their students to become full-fledged physicians and surgeons, their graduates faced difficult problems in being licensed as such. By 1937 only twenty-six legislatures had agreed to extend them privileges commensurate to those enjoyed by the M.D.'s, and in some of these states a majority of D.O.'s continued to be ineligible since sixteen mandated preprofessional college work and eight stipulated a year-long internship.[32] Furthermore, even when these requirements were met, other hurdles remained. In those jurisdictions where D.O.'s had to be examined before medical or composite boards, they fared rather poorly on the same written tests taken by allopathic candidates. Between 1927 and 1931, for example, only 48 percent passed compared to 95 percent of the M.D.'s.[33] Consequently, many D.O.'s avoided these examinations altogether, choosing an unlimited-license state whose tests were devised and graded by an osteopathic board and where the rate of failure was negligible. This reinforced the disproportionate geographical distribution of D.O.'s that had existed since early in the century and that had been directly related to the location of the colleges.[34]

Unable to convince the legislatures to eliminate independent osteopathic boards, the M.D.'s adopted the strategy of lobbying for a common test in the basic sciences that was to be taken prior to an actual licensing examination. This preliminary exam, required of all health care practitioners, would cover such subjects as anatomy, physiology, bacteriology, and pathology, and would be written and administered by a separate committee. In 1925 Connecticut and Wisconsin became the first to create basic science boards, followed by Minnesota, Nebraska, and Washington two years later.[35] In opposing such measures, the AOA House of Delegates argued, "Such an arrangement creates superfluous and unnecessary machinery of administration, erects another financial barrier to the recent graduate who is starting upon his life's work of helping the suffering; is an inadequate practical test in the fundamental subjects considering the varying viewpoints and methods of the different schools of practice; eliminates reciprocity between existing osteopathic boards which are now functioning in a manner to insure the public osteopathic physicians who are well qualified and furnishes the opportunity for domination by so-called 'regular medicine.'"[36] Their real fear, however, was that their graduates would not be able to do as well as the allopaths, and this was soon confirmed by early results. In 1930 before seven basic science boards the pass rate was 88.3 percent for M.D.'s, 54.5 percent for D.O.'s, and 21.9 percent for chiropractors.[37] As a consequence, osteopaths also began avoiding these exams. One AOA spokesman noted, "In the three states, Minnesota, Nebraska and Washington where the figures are available to make such a comparison, we find that those states jointly licensed 158 D.O.'s in the two and one half year period prior to the adoption of the basic science boards. In the two and one half year period since . . . they have licensed but 35 or about one-fifth as many."[38]

In accounting for their mediocre performance on basic science as well as medical board tests, the D.O.'s asserted that they were being discriminated against, since osteopathic emphases were being ignored. If such examinations contained a fair number of questions bearing upon the mechanics of vertebral articulations or upon the role of the nerves in controlling physiological functions, they argued, the results would be quite different.[39] This claim may have had some validity; however, it seems unlikely that these alleged biases were all that significant in contributing to the osteopaths' rate of failure. A more likely reason can be found in the simple fact that the M.D.'s as a group had a superior overall educational background than they did.

With almost one-half of the states refusing to grant D.O.'s unlimited privileges, with an ever-increasing number of states setting preprofessional and postdoctoral requirements most graduates could not fulfill, and with D.O.'s doing so poorly on outside examinations, the schools recognized a need for fundamental change in the structure and quality of osteopathic education. A mere continuation of their slow evolutionary approach to reform was not likely to achieve the privileges they sought and could conceivably cause them to lose what legal ground they had already gained.

The specter of this second possibility was raised by a 1934 survey of four osteopathic schools made by two Canadian academicians, Frederick Etherington, M.D., and S. Stanley Ryerson, M.D., which had been prompted by D.O.'s in Ontario who sought additional practice rights. By comparing these osteopathic institutions with that province's three medical colleges, Etherington and Ryerson showed that the D.O. schools were characterized by inferior laboratories and equipment, smaller hospital and clinic facilities, lower matriculation requirements, and less qualified faculties. As osteopathic colleges did not, in their opinion, adequately prepare students to become physicians and surgeons, their graduates should not be licensed as such.[40] These findings and conclusions were widely publicized by the AMA, which brought this survey to the attention of United States lawmakers.[41] Put on the defensive, the D.O.'s maintained that this "so-called inspection" was hastily done, that the examiners were obviously prejudiced, and that much of the information published was either misleading or blatantly untrue.[42]

While some state representatives gave the D.O.'s the benefit of the doubt, others called for an unbiased legislative inquiry. As a few states appeared on the brink of authorizing such investigations, the Associated Colleges hired an outside consultant, L. E. Blauch, Ph.D., a nationally known educator who for the past several years had headed a Carnegie Foundation study of the curricula of American dental schools. In 1936 Blauch, with the approval and cooperation of the AOA, accompanied John E. Rogers, D.O., chairman of the Bureau of Professional Education, on his regular inspection of five osteopathic colleges to gather data for his own separate and confidential evaluation. If the D.O.'s were expecting a more favorable portrait of conditions within, they were sadly disappointed. In a detailed and dispassionate series of reports, Blauch cited the same deficiencies as those noted in the Canadian survey.[43] Obviously, should the legislatures decide to commission their own investigations, the legal status of the colleges would be placed in considerable jeopardy.

Where the M.D.'s made their largest strides in terms of standards in the first twenty-five years following the Flexner report, the D.O.'s made theirs during the second. One of the earliest reforms they effected was in pre-professional education requirements. In 1934 Philadelphia began enforcing a one year of college qualification, and in 1937 it followed Los Angeles, which twelve months earlier had increased its minimum to two years. Chicago and Kansas City went directly from a high school diploma to a two-year prerequisite in 1938, while Des Moines and Kirksville, meeting an AOA-imposed deadline, instituted a one-year condition in 1938 and a two-year in 1940.[44]

As anticipated, enrollment suffered. In 1937 there were 1,977 students in the six accredited colleges; by 1940 the number had dipped to 1,653, a decline of 21 percent. This trend was accelerated by the entry of the United States into the Second World War, which drastically reduced the number of individuals eligible to enter any professional school. In 1945 total osteopathic enrollment had shrunk to 556—by far its lowest point in the century.[45] Immediately after the war the AOA hired a full-time vocational counselor who visited liberal arts colleges across the country, meeting their placement officers and students, and acquainting them with osteopathy.[46] This campaign, in conjunctions with the schools' separate recruiting drives, which were aimed not only at current undergraduates but returning veterans as well, soon brought the desired results. In 1947 total matriculation had climbed back to its average prior to the establishment of the two-year prerequisite, and it remained stable for more than a decade. Indeed, during this period the ratio of qualified applicants to available freshman positions rose to roughly two to one, making admission into the colleges competitive for the first time.[47] This served to strengthen the credentials of osteopathic students and encouraged each of the schools—Los Angeles in 1949; Chicago, Des Moines, and Kansas City in 1952; and Kirksville and Philadelphia in 1954—to raise its mandatory minimum entrance requirement to three years of college work. By 1960, 70.9 percent of all new osteopathic students were entering with a bachelor's or an advanced degree.[48]

As higher prerequisites for admission were being introduced, osteopathic schools were enriching their basic science curriculum. Although the total combined average number of hours in anatomy, physiology, biochemistry, pathology, and microbiology remained virtually unchanged from 1935 and 1936 to 1948 and 1949, the percentage of time spent in the laboratory as opposed to the lecture hall jumped from 47.9 percent to 59.0 percent, a figure that continued to climb in subsequent years.[49] Three of the schools, Chicago, Kansas City, and Los Angeles, erected new basic science buildings, while the others upgraded existing facilities and equipment. Furthermore, after 1945 each of the colleges began hiring full-time instructors with M.S. and Ph.D. degrees, thereby enhancing the quality of their faculties.[50] An even greater transformation occurred in the other half of the osteopathic curriculum. Actual bedside and outpatient experience for each student was increased in the six schools from an average of 862 hours in academic year 1935-36, to 1,883 hours in 1948-49, to 2,214 in 1958-59.[51] This can be attributed both to the expansion of the college hospitals from a combined total of 530 beds and bassinets in 1935 to 1,344 in 1959, and to the fact that each of the schools made arrangements with other osteopathic hospitals for the training of externs.[52]

Quite a few of these changes in undergraduate education were possible only because the schools set themselves in a more financially secure position. Since the annual number of qualified applicants far exceeded the freshman places available, the colleges could institute sizable tuition boosts without jeopardizing the number of matriculants. Between 1935 and 1960 fees climbed from an average of $223 to $900 per year.[53] Outside sources were also solicited. In 1943 the AOA launched what became known as the Osteopathic Progress Fund. With student enrollment then dropping to dangerously low levels and with several of the schools faced with the prospect of having to close their doors, D.O.'s in the field were pressured to contribute. By mid-1944, at the end of the first campaign, an impressive total of $962,535 was subscribed and directly channeled into the college treasuries.[54] In 1946 a new, continuous, Osteopathic Progress Fund program was organized which raised $8,956,625 between then and 1961.[55] This era also marked the genesis of federal support. In 1951 the United States Public Health Service awarded all six schools renewable teaching grants previously designated for M.D. and dental colleges. By 1956 this source of income amounted to $383,000 a year. Another federal program aiding the schools came in the form of hospital construction funds made possible under the Hill Burton Act of 1946.[56] Among the major grants made prior to 1960 was one awarded to Kansas City for a new clinic, one to Kirksville for a modern inpatient facility, and a third to Los Angeles for a rehabilitation center.

The advances in predoctoral education during this period were accompanied by significant changes on the postgraduate level. In 1936 the AOA Bureau of Hospitals undertook its first inspection of institutions offering internships. Since the primary objective of the association was to provide a position for every new graduate, requirements were initially set low in order to qualify as many of their hospitals as possible.[57] During the Second World War the D.O.'s, who as a group were exempt from the draft and had been declared ineligible for voluntary service with the military medical corps, began taking care of the clients of inducted M.D.'s. With allopathic hospitals still refusing them admitting and staff privileges, their new patients helped underwrite the costs of building and maintaining separate private osteopathic institutions. In 1945 there were approximately 260 D.O. hospitals operating in the country, more than tripling the total of a decade earlier.[58] This in turn served to alleviate the internship shortage, and by 1951 available positions had surpassed the number of that year's graduating seniors, thus making possible the toughening of standards.[59] In 1947 the Bureau of Hospitals

### TABLE 1
M.D., D.O., and Chriopractor
Basic Science Board Examination Results, 1942-44 to 1951-53

| Period | M.D. Examinees | | | D.O. Examinees | | | Chiropractic Examinees | | |
|--------|----------|--------|------|----------|--------|------|----------|--------|------|
| | Examined | Passed | % | Examined | Passed | % | Examined | Passed | % |
| 1942-44 | 6,339 | 5,442 | 85.8 | 545 | 285 | 52.2 | 59 | 23 | 38.9 |
| 1945-47 | 8,628 | 6,935 | 80.3 | 526 | 306 | 58.1 | 134 | 41 | 30.5 |
| 1948-50 | 8,921 | 7,768 | 87.0 | 1,032 | 629 | 60.9 | 1,489 | 224 | 35.1 |
| 1951-53 | 9,693 | 8,448 | 87.1 | 903 | 723 | 80.0 | 579 | 217 | 37.4 |

*Source:* "Medical Licensure Statistics," *Journal of the American Medical Association* 122 (1943): 111; 125 (1944): 143; 128 (1945): 123; 131 (1946): 133; 134 (1947): 283; 137 (1948): 638; 140 (1949): 321; 143 (1950): 471; 146 (1951): 372; 149 (1952): 479; 152 (1953): 450; 155 (1954): 482. Beginning in 1954 results by type of practitioner were not reported.

### TABLE 2
United States-Trained M.D. and D.O. Physicians and Foreign Medical Graduates
Examination Results before Medical and Composite Licensing Boards, 1940-44 to 1955-59

| Period | U.S. M.D. Examinees | | | U.S. D.O. Examinees | | | Foreign Medical Graduates | | |
|--------|----------|--------|------|----------|--------|------|----------|--------|------|
| | Examined | Passed | % | Examined | Passed | % | Examined | Passed | % |
| 1940-44 | 27,158 | 26,291 | 96.8 | 940 | 589 | 62.6 | 7,152 | 3,371 | 47.1 |
| 1945-49 | 26,840 | 26,005 | 96.8 | 881 | 618 | 70.1 | 2,943 | 1,339 | 45.4 |
| 1950-54 | 27,052 | 26,145 | 96.6 | 1,021 | 810 | 79.3 | 6,118 | 3,270 | 53.4 |
| 1955-59 | 30,184 | 28,903 | 95.7 | 1,174 | 954 | 81.2 | 11,192 | 6,787 | 60.6 |

*Sources:* D.O. figures from 1940 to 1945 were culled from "Report of the American Association of Osteopathic Examiners: 1952," microfilmed, American Osteopathic Association Archives, Chicago. Subsequent D.O. data and all M.D. information derived from "Medical Licensure Statistics," *Journal of the American Medical Association* 116 (1941): 2025; 119 (1942): 145; 122 (1943): 94; 125 (1944): 126; 128 (1945): 106; 131 (1946): 114; 134 (1947): 260; 137 (1948): 609; 140 (1949): 298; 143 (1950): 446; 146 (1951): 344; 149 (1952): 450; 152 (1953): 421; 155 (1954): 452; 158 (1955): 275; 161 (1956): 341; 164 (1957): 426; 167 (1958): 573; 170 (1959): 573; 173 (1960): 387.
*Note:* Osteopathic data include candidates from both AOA-accredited and nonaccredited schools. U.S. M.D. data reflect those graduates from AMA-accredited institutions only.

made its first inspection of osteopathic residency programs. That year, 71 were approved; by 1959 there were 389 available.[60] As formal residencies increased in number, the requirements governing them, as well as the process of certification of specialists (under machinery created by the AOA in 1939),[61] were considerably strengthened.

The push for higher standards between 1935 and 1960 resulted in progress on the legal front. At the end of this span of time, the number of states in which D.O.'s became eligible for unlimited licensure rose to thirty-eight;

osteopathic schools were now able to meet the requirements of certain medical boards and other governmental agencies which had been empowered to approve them; and D.O. graduates possessed a preprofessional background and postgraduate training matching or exceeding the minimum called for by each state.[62]

Osteopathic performance on outside examinations also showed significant gains. While from 1942-44 to 1951-53 results obtained by M.D.'s and chiropractors on basic science tests remained virtually unchanged, the D.O.'s went from a 52.2 percent to an 80.0 percent pass rate (table 1). Substantial increases were also made before state medical and composite boards of licensure. Here too, while the results of United States medical graduates remained constant from 1940-44 to 1955-59, the rate of passage for D.O.'s climbed from 62.6 percent to 81.2 percent (table 2). Clearly, whatever educational problems remained, the D.O.'s had placed their academic house upon a more solid foundation.

# CHAPTER SEVEN

# A Question
# of Identity

Osteopathy as originally conceived by Andrew Still was a radically different approach to healing. Its philosophy, view of pathology, and system of patient care shared little with the components of orthodox medicine. Indeed, the founder cast himself and his followers as nothing less than revolutionaries seeking to overturn the entrenched allopathic order. However, as the D.O.'s came to adopt a multidimensional conception of disease and as their scope broadened, the objective differences between the two groups began to fade. This trend would later be accelerated by two further developments: first, the progress made in improving their standards as just described; and second, by their growing reliance upon orthodox medical modalities. However, these transformations were not accompanied by a commensurate change in the general public's perception of who the osteopathic practitioner was and what he did. As a result, most D.O.'s would suffer, to varying degrees, from status inconsistency.

### The Displacement of Osteopathic Manipulative Therapy

The one feature of osteopathic practice that most readily distinguished the D.O.'s from the M.D.'s was, of course, manipulative therapy. After 1930, however, the application of this modality in total patient management began a steady decline. This trend can be attributed to, first, institutional changes, that is, alterations in the social structure of the colleges, the hospitals, and office practice; and second, to scientific changes, that is, transformations in the D.O.'s' knowledge base.

The improvements that were undertaken in the colleges beginning in the 1930s were all initiated with the idea of raising their graduates' chances of becoming eligible for and passing unlimited licensure examinations. Since the distinctive elements of osteopathic education had no specific relevance to these goals, the colleges had no incentive to emphasize or build up this area of the course. Indeed, some of the improvements were often instituted at the expense of distinctive osteopathy. Many of the full-time non-D.O.

teachers hired to upgrade the standards of basic science instruction, for example, did not have the background necessary to integrate osteopathic theory into their lectures, as their predecessors had.[1] Also, the time spent on pharmacology and surgery was increased to meet state requirements, and this seemed to have a detrimental effect with regard to osteopathic instruction. The consequence, complained G. W. Woodbury, D.O. of Los Angeles, was that too many students were becoming "sadly confused and sorely disillusioned before their day of graduation. . . . The lavish display of therapeutic methods and modalities explained and utilized in college, hospital and clinic demonstrations has a tendency to weaken the emphasis on and minimize the need and value of distinctly osteopathic procedures."[2]

In the first osteopathic hospitals, the admitting D.O. would perform the surgery himself or at the very least handle the patient's pre- and postoperative manipulative care. However, with the advent of larger facilities and the establishment of a more clear-cut division of labor between the hospital-based and office-based physician, the D.O. general practitioner was less involved in such management. As a result, osteopathic manipulative therapy (O.M.T.) waned. Besides claiming that they were "too busy" to administer such treatment themselves, more and more full-time D.O. surgeons viewed it as impractical from a technical standpoint, particularly when the patient was in an oxygen tent, or hooked up to assorted monitors and intravenous lines. Indeed, many D.O. surgeons argued on these grounds alone that O.M.T. was only suitable in ambulatory settings.[3]

This deemphasis and growing exclusion of O.M.T. from the hospitals had a significant impact upon the colleges' postdoctoral programs. In his 1946 AOA presidential address, C. Robert Starks, referring to their students, cited a fellow practitioner who complained, "As soon as these individuals are graduated and put into osteopathic hospitals they are immediately 'deosteopathized' [so] that by the time they finish their internships the osteopathic phase of their training has been discredited in large measure by osteopathic surgeons and other members of the staff, and those individuals go into practice with an apologetic attitude towards the osteopathic phase of their professional work."[4] Needless to say, accepting the accuracy of this generalization, the graduates who went on past the internship to take hospital-based residencies were even more likely to develop a negative opinion of O.M.T.

After the war the AOA Bureau of Professional Education and the Committee on Hospitals began to respond to this criticism. In 1947 the latter announced it would start enforcing a policy in effect since the beginning of the AOA accreditation program that house staff record distinctive osteopathic diagnostic and therapeutic procedures on all patient charts. The hospitals offered little cooperation, however, and within five years the advocates of enforcement were labeling their own efforts a failure.[5]

Institutional changes at the level of office-based D.O.'s were also affecting O.M.T. use. With the shift from an essentially chronic to a broad-based practice, the number of individuals daily seeking osteopathic office services steadily increased; the increased demand served to reduce the frequency and length of osteopathic treatments. To make more efficient use of their time, some practitioners turned to other physical modalities that did not require their continued presence, such as the spinalator, a device that could be automatically set to manipulate vertebrae mechanically. However, to a far larger number of D.O.'s, pharmacotherapy was a much more convenient substitute. The efficiency of writing a prescription or giving an injection over administering O.M.T. appears to have been, in itself, a significant factor in a D.O.'s decision on how he or she would manage a given patient.[6] Also critical in this regard were the patients' expectations on how they should be treated. Clients not previously socialized into the traditional osteopathic approach were less likely to expect or desire O.M.T. in disorders not directly involving the musculoskeletal system.[7]

As noted, scientific issues also impacted on the relative frequency of O.M.T. Early basic research, the bulk of which was carried out by Louisa Burns and her associates, lacked valid controls and for all practical purposes was worthless in regard to demonstrating that the lesion played any direct or indirect role in the pathogenesis of visceral disease. Indeed, some D.O.'s came to feel that in many illnesses the presence or absence of the lesion was irrelevant. In 1916, during the fight over the relative merits of the diphtheria antitoxin, Henry Bunting, editor of the *Osteopathic Physician,* asked his colleagues:

> Would we rather hang to our dogma that—no matter what the facts show—*it has always got to be a mechanical lesion?* Nothing is easier to prove in the case of diphtheria, at least, that the word "mechanical" has no business to be inserted as a necessary condition for getting that disease. The exciting cause is *vital,* not *mechanical*—the Klebs-Loeffler bacillus. Inject 100 guinea pigs, each of 250 grams weight, with an equal amount each (or 1-100th part) of minimum lethal dose of diphtheria toxin. Each guinea pig will be "sure dead" in 96 hours. Repeat the experiment with 1000 guinea pigs, the thousand will die. Repeat it with 1,000,000. The million will die on the same schedule. Does this mean anything? What caused the disease? What killed? Some unknown and different anatomical lesion in the case of each guinea pig, or the well known Klebs-Loeffler bacillus through its toxins.[8]

Carefully controlled research on the lesion under osteopathic auspices began in the late 1930s as a byproduct of the search by the profession for philanthropic support of its schools. J. Stedman Denslow, D.O., then at the Chicago College, met with Alan Gregg, Ph.D., of the Rockefeller Foundation, who advised that outside funding might be more readily secured if the D.O.'s scientifically demonstrated that they had a distinctive contribution to make to the healing arts. Through Gregg's help, Denslow, who had decided he would prepare himself for a research career, was introduced to a number of prominent neurophysiologists. Among those who provided him with counsel and assistance were Ralph Waldo Gerard, M.D., Ph.D., of the University of Chicago, and Detlev Bronk, Ph.D., of the University of Pennsylvania, both leaders in the new field of electromyography.[9]

Moving to Kirksville after he built one of the early differential amplifiers and recorders for simultaneous electromyographic observations of paravertebral musculature, Denslow launched his research. Unlike Burns, he purposefully confined himself to asking limited, testable questions regarding the lesion phenomena, particularly what local neurophysiological manifestations were associated with those spinal areas designated as lesioned through palpation. Between 1941 and 1943 Denslow and his associates published four articles in two prominent nonosteopathic basic scientific journals, demonstrating that the motor neurons (anterior horn cells) at those segmental levels in the spinal cord associated with musculoskeletal stress had lower reflex thresholds than those at other, "normal," levels in the spinal cord. This was shown by applying measured amounts of pressure necessary to evoke contractions of the paravertebral muscles at that segmental level. These muscular contractions were detailed and recorded electromyographically. He further found that reflex motor thresholds of the paravertebral muscles, that is to say, their motor neurons, differed at different levels of the trunk, and that the reflex thresholds for both muscle contraction and pain were low in lesion areas as compared to nonlesion or normal areas.[10]

After the Second World War Denslow was joined in his work by Irwin M. Korr, a Ph.D. from the University of Pennsylvania. Continuing this general line of experimentation, the two men demonstrated in 1947 that diffuse and remote stimuli from many sources preferentially excited the motor neurons of lesioned segments while nonlesioned segments remained quiescent. The results of this investigation, added to the data from Denslow's previous work, indicated that the neurogenic mechanism responsible for this phenomenon was facilitation (that is, reduced threshold of excitability) of the motor neurons of the spinal cord. Although the source of the facilitation was not at that time conclusively demonstrated, it was hypothesized that it might have its origin in a sustained afferent muscle bombardment from segmentally related somatic or visceral structures. These impulses would have the effect of lowering the threshold of excitability of the neurons at the segmental level in the spinal cord's associated stress area.[11]

This research effort at Kirksville, which has continued for decades, was of great import to the profession. It provided the first objective evidence of the presence of what the D.O.'s had designated through palpation as the "osteopathic lesion"; it showed that a D.O. could do reputable studies on the lesion phenomenon and have the results accepted by the outside sci-

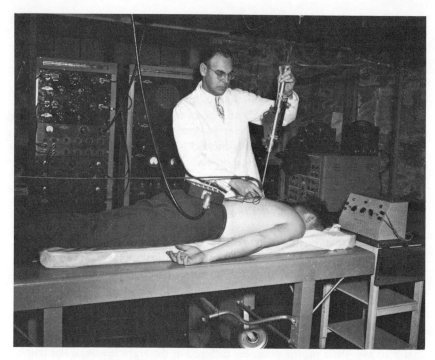

*J. S. Denslow, D.O., conducting electromyographic research
(early 1950s). Courtesy of Dr. Denslow.*

entific community; and it paved the way for federal support of osteopathic research. However, the investigations, while breaking new ground, could not resolve two key questions. First, what was the significance of the lesion in the etiology of disease? Second, what effect, if any, would the elimination of the lesion through manipulation have on the disease process?

To some extent controlled clinical research on manipulation might have been able to resolve this second issue; however, no such studies were undertaken in this era. The failure to pursue this course can be attributed in large part to serious methodological difficulties inherent in this type of project. Though one could easily standardize the content and strength of a pill, it would be most difficult to have the same control over the amplitude and velocity of physical manipulation. Furthermore, it was relatively simple to set up a single or double blind study with a capsule. Neither the patient nor the doctor would be able to distinguish the test drug from the placebo. However, what would constitute a manipulative placebo? The fact that one could not easily eliminate the subjective element from clinical studies on manipulation convinced those D.O.'s within the AOA who controlled limited association funding for scientific projects to place their energy and money in basic research.[12] The clinical investigations that were carried out and published in osteopathic journals consisted of a small number of case studies, many of which were anecdotal in content. Thus D.O.'s were told by their colleagues that the lesion was significant and that O.M.T. worked, but they had to accept the concepts on faith or on circumstantial evidence. A growing number could not. As Louis Chandler, D.O. of Los Angeles, noted in 1950, "Too much still seems to be in the realm of uncertainty both as to what will result from manipulation in the area of the spinal vertebral lesion and in the physiological consequences [elsewhere]. . . . These uncertainties constitute a great obstacle to many scientifically trained men in maintaining an interest in osteopathy. Uncertainty regarding an observation to them means that it probably is not valid."[13]

While clinical research in distinctive osteopathic procedures was standing still, the value of new chemotherapeutic discoveries was steadily being demonstrated. In 1935 the first of the synthetically produced sulfonamides useful against hemolytic streptococci and staphylococci was introduced. Early in the 1940s penicillin, effective against the range of gram positive bacteria, became available. Beginning in 1945 streptomycin, which destroyed gram negative bacteria, was marketed. This was followed by aureomycin, the first of the broad spectrum antibiotics, and soon afterward by chloramphenicol and tetracycline. In addition to these antibiotics, a number of new analgesics, anti-inflammatory agents, muscle relaxants, tranquilizers, as well as other forms of chemotherapy were introduced prior to 1960.[14] Where the drug manufacturers could provide tangible (if not always reliable) statistical evidence supporting the value and safety of their products, the advocates of O.M.T. could offer little more than testimonials. As a result, Chandler's "scientifically" trained D.O. was more likely to put greater trust in these modalities than in manipulation.

The relative decline in dependence on O.M.T. over the years is imperfectly reflected in the changing focus of the *JAOA*. In the early 1930s O.M.T. was still included in the majority of articles and was described with great care and detail, but by 1948 the AOA Board of Trustees felt compelled to pass a resolution urging that "every effort be made by the writers of scientific papers for publication in the official Journal of the Association or in other osteopathic periodicals to include wherever feasible discussion of the relationship of the osteopathic concept to the subject of the paper."[15] However, as the contributors were increasingly specialists who had eschewed structural diagnosis and manipulative therapy in their own practice, this resolution had little if any impact. By the end of the 1950s most *JAOA* articles failed to mention O.M.T., and when they did it was only briefly and more as an adjunct than as an integral part of patient management. Articles devoted solely to osteopathic principles would still appear, but with far less frequency.[16]

Those D.O.'s who strongly believed in the appropriateness of O.M.T. in a wide range of conditions did what they could to alter this trend. In 1938 a group calling itself the Osteopathic Manipulative Therapeutic and Clinical Research Association, which after 1944 was renamed the Academy of Applied Osteopathy, was granted affiliate status with the AOA. The academy arranged programs covering osteopathic principles and practice at the national AOA conventions, circulated papers to members, provided speakers for state and local AOA meetings, conducted short postgraduate refresher courses, and sponsored the writing or distribution of books relating to distinctive osteopathic approaches. While keeping traditional osteopathy before the profession, the influence of the academy was limited. Only 12 percent of all D.O.'s in the AOA were affiliated with the academy group at its peak.[17]

Precisely how many D.O.'s in the 1950s were performing manipulation and to what extent is impossible to determine, although one can come to certain general conclusions. Hospital-based D.O.'s were utilizing O.M.T. infrequently, and only a minority of surgeons saw to it that their patients received pre- and postoperative treatments. In office-based general practice, O.M.T. still appears to have been used with some regularity, but less time was devoted to it and it was increasingly restricted to the treatment of local joint and muscle problems. While approximately 10 percent of all active D.O.'s, either through choice or because of state laws, were then confining themselves to distinctive osteopathic procedures, this group (comprised mostly of older D.O.'s) was steadily shrinking each year. As for younger practitioners, the data are more substantial. In 1954 the AOA mailed out a confidential questionnaire to all active D.O.'s who graduated between 1948 and 1953. Close to 60 percent responded. Only 44 percent of those answering the question, "What percentage of your patients receive manipulative therapy?" said over 50 percent. Considerable variation by school was noted; 53 percent of Kirksville graduates responded with this figure, compared to 16 percent of Los Angeles graduates.[18] Clearly the D.O.'s as a group were coming continually closer to the M.D. in terms of patient management.

## Status Inconsistency

The most vexing problem for the D.O.'s as they expanded their scope of practice and improved their educational standards was that of public non-recognition of the complete range of services they could provide their clients, with a concomitant lesser deference and social standing than that accorded the M.D. To the many D.O.'s who believed themselves as well trained or as competent as their allopathic counterparts, these circumstances led to considerable frustration and alienation.

Part of their difficulty lay in their small numbers. From the turn of the century up through 1960, the D.O.'s constituted approximately 5 percent of the total United States physician population (M.D. and D.O. totals combined). Furthermore, as previously noted, the D.O.'s were distributed disproportionately, and in many sections of the country an individual could not obtain osteopathic care. Indeed, as late as 1960, twenty-two states had fewer than fifty D.O.'s apiece. This helped to make the profession socially invisible.[19]

Another handicap preventing widespread approval or recognition was their difficulty in securing the same legal privileges as those accorded the M.D.'s. This applied not only to unlimited licensure laws, but to winning the right to handle workmen's compensation cases, becoming state or local health officials, entering the military medical corps, gaining access to public hospitals, and having their services covered under private insurance plans sanctioned by special enabling acts. Not having any or all of these rights served "officially" to brand the D.O.'s as inferior practitioners.

Because of these various circumstances many, perhaps most, Americans were unclear as to who the D.O. was and what precisely he or she did. In 1936 the AOA hired a public relations counselor who conducted several man-on-the-street interviews in downtown Chicago. To the question "What is an osteopath?" a magazine writer responded, "An osteopath is a fellow who sets your spine, an M.D. who specializes in that method." A women's clothing stylist answered, "He's a man who has something to do with the spine." A bus driver declared, "Well, I don't know if I can word it. He massages people." A postal clerk replied, "An osteopath has something to do with care of the feet?" Another postal clerk replied, "An osteopath has something to do with massage like a chiropractor. Osteopaths I believe are outlawed in New York and some other states too. I read about some of them being arrested in New York." A department store clerk exclaimed, "Oh yes, I know. I went to one once. They are especially for nervous people and treat them by massaging." A department store manager observed, "The difference between a doctor and an osteopath is that an osteopath is drugless." A policeman reflected, "Let's see. He's a guy that when somebody gets all bent up, they put him on a table and twist him around and sorta put him together again. Ain't that right?" And finally, a stockbroker remarked, "He's a man who lays you on a table and massages. A doctor can be an osteopath but an osteopath can't be a doctor."[20] While these beliefs were expressed in what was then a limited practice state, the situation in unlimited or nearly unlimited states was not much better. During the same year Professor George Hartmann of Columbia University published a study of the relative social status of twenty-five medical careers as judged by 250 Pennsylvania laymen. The category "osteopath" was ranked eighteenth overall, one notch below "dietician."[21]

The profession acted in a number of ways to change its image. The first effort, which gained some momentum in the 1920s, concerned the matter of occupational title. Because the term *osteopath* had been so closely identified with manipulative therapy, it was believed new labels were needed. L. Alice Foley, D.O., writing in the *JAOA,* related the story of an attorney who said to her, "'Now you osteopaths do so and so, but the physician does thus and so.' The thought came to me that the public does differentiate. They call the allopath their physician and think of us as osteopaths." Foley recommended the use of the term *osteopathic physician.* "That explains the kind of physician we are, and it also leaves the word 'physician' in their thoughts concerning us." M. F. Hulett, D.O., agreed, stating that "many of our friends are not yet aware of the fact that we are physicians at all, and some still seem surprised that we really treat the sick." Commenting upon "osteopathic physician" and "osteopathic physician and surgeon," Hulett added, "I am quite sure the repeated use of these terms will add to the dignity of our school." This move received support from then-AOA editor Cyrus Gaddis, D.O., who sermonized: "Let no piece of literature be circulated or none go out with simply 'osteopath.' Let it stand out 'osteopathic physician' and then be sure that we are ready to live up to that name. . . . Are you an osteopathic physician or just an osteopath? Times are changing. Are we willing to have the public consider us simple treatment givers?"[22] By 1940 all but a small number of D.O.'s were using the new labels.

Concurrent with the move by D.O.'s to modify their shingles and office stationery, the national and state associations sought to bring up to date those references to *osteopathy* found in dictionaries and encyclopedias. Phrases or definitions which suggested that D.O.'s were not in favor of drugs, or that they placed chief attention in their work upon finding and removing structural lesions through manipulation, were excised in favor of language that emphasized that osteopathy was a complete school of healing.[23] Telephone directory listings were also altered, substituting *osteopathic physician* or *osteopathic physician and surgeon,* depending on the licensure law, for the now-discredited word *osteopath.*[24]

The AOA, as described in part elsewhere, also worked to improve the D.O.'s' social standing through the legislatures and the courts. As a result, many licensure laws would be revised in their favor; D.O.'s became included in some of the health-related New Deal programs; they would win attorney general and judicial decisions on their participation in workmen's compensation cases; they triumphed in some key battles over their right to access to hospitals built with public money; and they qualified for some federal aid, mostly in the form of Hill-Burton grants.[25]

All of these efforts helped to improve the D.O.'s' public image through the 1950s, but the rate of progress for many of them was far from satisfactory. One of the principal reasons for their failure to make larger inroads lay in their inability to convince the print media to spread the osteopathic message. National and state conventions, as well as D.O. speaker tours, were not considered particularly noteworthy, and when such events were reported, the resulting story was usually no more than a few paragraphs in length and was placed in an inconspicuous section of the newspaper. Most national general feature magazines also seemed to see little of interest in the profession, and those that did focused entirely upon the manipulative aspect. Typical was Mark Sullivan's "If I Need Relaxation," published in the *Reader's Digest,* an article that, while most complimentary, cast the D.O.'s as highly skilled "rubbers" rather than broadly trained physicians, thus reinforcing the image the movement wanted to shed.[26]

When newspapers and magazines gave prominent attention to the activities of individual M.D.'s, it was often in connection with the introduction of a new drug or a new life-saving surgical technique, or the reception of a prestigious award. Other M.D.'s were regularly featured in periodicals by contributing health columns. The D.O.'s, the great majority of whom were in the unglamorous field of general practice and made no spectacular contribution to research, were thus cut off from such favorable coverage. Indeed, when reporters focused on the exploits of certain osteopathic practitioners, it was almost invariably connected with alleged or actual deviant behavior: a botched operation, an injury related to manipulation, an illegal abortion, a quack cure, or the like.[27] When M.D.'s were charged with similar malpractice, the public, given its knowledge of the medical profession as a whole, could dismiss these as isolated instances. However, because the same public had little or no prior knowledge of osteopathy, the activities of a few could be easily generalized to characterize the abilities or behavior of all D.O.'s.

This continued lack of public awareness of who the D.O. was and what he did generated a considerable degree of frustration among many members of the profession. Although most practitioners simply accepted the fact that a certain portion of their work consisted of answering questions relating to how much educational training they received, what their scope of practice was, and how precisely they differed from the M.D., other D.O.'s found this situation intolerable. This problem of poor public perception carried over to affect the D.O.'s family as well. During social interaction, wives and children were always at risk of being put into the uncomfortable or embarrassing position of having to explain or even defend their spouse's or parent's occupation. In 1955 AOA editor Raymond Keesecker, addressing the student doctor's wife, noted that such situations "Give you the best opportunity in the world for some important public relations work." However, some wives saw this as a terrible burden, and even Keesecker noted that in dealing with any question about osteopathy, "it is not too easy to give a specific answer."[28]

Many D.O.'s came to believe that the primary cause of their identity problem were the letters behind their names. The American public, they argued, recognized the M.D. degree as the universal symbol for a physician and surgeon; thus it was not all that surprising that patients seeing any other designation would be confused as to its meaning, even if *physician and surgeon* were added. In their opinion, the easiest way of changing their image was to change the degree awarded by osteopathic colleges to that of M.D. During the 1920s and 1930s, such calls were occasionally sounded in the journals, but they gained no support within organized osteopathy as a whole.[29] However, with America on the verge of entering the Second World War, the administrations of two of the schools were besieged by many students and alumni to adopt the M.D. designation in the belief that through this maneuver they could become eligible to serve their country as military physicians. To take the onus off the school officials and put an end to such unrealistic hopes, the AOA Board of Trustees in 1941 declared that "the only degree to be issued by an approved osteopathic college qualifying for licensure to practice the healing art shall be the degree of doctor of osteopathy."[30] As far as the AOA was concerned, this decision was absolute and irrevocable.

The refusal by the AOA to accommodate this dissatisfied minority led some to obtain diploma-mill M.D. degrees to hang in their offices. Such certificates, while totally worthless for the purpose of licensure, were nonetheless thought useful by their possessors as a means of convincing new patients that they were after all "real doctors."[31] However, a larger group of unhappy practitioners were not willing to go that far. They simply decided to leave all mention of their D.O. degree and reference to osteopathy off their stationery and shingle and just go by the title "Dr. 'so and so', Physician and Surgeon."[32] Thus, while the public was confused as to the identity of the D.O.'s, a significant number of osteopathic practitioners were coming to the conclusion that the best way to deal with their problems was to confuse it even further.

# CHAPTER EIGHT

# *The California Merger*

For most D.O.'s the problems connected with their identity did not undermine the desire for professional autonomy. Even many of those who failed to advertise themselves as osteopathic practitioners and favored the schools awarding an M.D. degree continued to believe they were part of a distinctive group that should remain politically separate and independent. Their displeasure with the AOA was with its policy, not its legitimacy as the voice of osteopathy. However, this attitude was not universally shared. For some D.O.'s the various changes taking place within the profession, combined with their specific situation at the local level, led to a vastly different interpretation and outlook. Nowhere was this more evident or widespread than in California.

## The COA and the CMA

In the decades prior to 1960 there were more D.O.'s practicing in California than in any other state, constituting at any given time 10 percent of all its physicians, with perhaps 15 percent of its total population as their patients.[1] In terms of legislative victories, public acceptance, and average income, no other state group approached their achievements; however, a deep disenchantment with their lot belied their outward success.

Even before the turn of the century California D.O.'s were beginning to establish themselves as the progressive wing of osteopathy. In 1896 the Pacific College became the first school to introduce a mandatory two-year course and later was one of the earliest to expand to three years. The state attracted and became the stronghold for the "broad osteopaths," and under their influence the Los Angeles College became the first institution to place in its curriculum an ongoing course in *materia medica*. In the realm of preprofessional standards, the College of Osteopathic Physicians and Surgeons (COP&S) — the result of combining the aforementioned schools — was the first to insist upon one year, then two years, and ultimately three years of prior college work as an entrance requirement. Finally, with respect to clinical facilities, it was the first and only school to utilize a large municipal hospital for bedside and outpatient teaching.

Pointing with pride to these various innovations and achievements, California D.O.'s generally regarded themselves as the best qualified osteopathic physicians and surgeons in the country. Many also considered themselves the most "scientific," which meant the decline in distinctive osteopathy was more pronounced in California than elsewhere. Furthermore, because of the stringent requirements of California law as well as tougher regulations adopted by the state board of osteopathic examiners, graduates from other D.O. schools were for many years ineligible for unrestricted licenses. This made for a comparatively homogeneous osteopathic population.

California D.O.'s early on placed a high priority on securing complete equality with the M.D.'s in their state. It was thus a source of continuing frustration for them that whatever progress they collectively made, significant gaps between the two groups remained. This was reflected most clearly in the matter of college finances. From the 1930s through the early 1960s, COP&S could spend perhaps only one-half to three-fifths of the funds allocated by M.D. schools for the education of each student, since it could not count upon state support, general university funds, and foundation philanthropy. Thus, although it was consistently able to employ more full-time faculty than other osteopathic colleges, COP&S could not approach the numbers characteristic of an AMA-accredited institution.[2]

Far worse was their postgraduate situation, particularly with respect to training facilities for residents. Only a small number of positions were available annually within the entire state, and all but a few of these were offered at a single institution, Los Angeles County Osteopathic Hospital. While several dozen other D.O. facilities were founded in California after 1930, the bed capacity of the great majority was too limited to provide for an adequate specialty program. Those applicants not successfully placed had to either go out of state or resign themselves to a general practice. At the same time, the D.O.'s could only look with envy at the number of quality allopathic hospital residencies in their midst, appointments for which they as osteopathic physicians were ineligible.

Added to these educational problems was that of publicity. Public knowledge about the D.O.'s, particularly the scope of their services, was still far less than what was known of the M.D.'s, in spite of the fact that a significant minority of the California population was served by D.O.'s. Part of this problem was attributed to the continuous waves of new residents arriving from other areas of the country where the profession had far fewer representatives and limited practice rights. Some California D.O.'s argued that in one sense they were being victimized by the national image of osteopathy and held the AOA responsible, alleging that it was too tolerant of the lower standards maintained by the other colleges and was not working hard enough to eliminate remaining legal and social inequalities.[3]

This combination of elements—namely a group of D.O.'s thinking of themselves as a breed apart from the rest, along with the other problems which faced the profession generally, such as poorer educational opportunities, lack of public recognition, and a decline in the use of distinctive osteopathic procedures—led an increasing number of California practitioners to consider seriously the possibility and advantages of leaving organized osteopathy for organized medicine.

While more California D.O.'s were coming to this conclusion, so too were the leaders of the state's medical association, but for entirely different reasons. For the most part, organized medicine within California saw the D.O.'s as an inferior group of practitioners who were lowering the general quality of health care in the state. For decades they had tried through various legislative means to eliminate the profession, but to no avail. Despite their small number, the D.O.'s had been able to wield considerable political power, effectively blocking the passage of threatening measures. With no other viable strategy left open to them, the M.D.'s gradually came to believe that the only way to destroy osteopathy was through the absorption of the D.O.'s, much as the homeopaths and eclectics had been swallowed up early in the century.[4]

In 1943 Forest Grunigan, D.O., president of the California Osteopathic Association (COA), appointed an official Fact-Finding Committee to meet with representatives of the California Medical Association (CMA) as the culmination of informal contacts concerning merger that had begun five years earlier.[5] At this meeting the CMA offered a proposal for amalgamation which they had already discussed with the AMA Council on Medical Education and the Association of American Medical Colleges. This plan called for: (1) the granting of M.D. degrees to all D.O.'s licensed as physicians and surgeons in California by one of the existing four medical schools in the state; (2) the elimination of the osteopathic licensing boards; and (3) conversion of COP&S into a medical school. Since neither the council nor the Association of American Medical Colleges had yet approved the plan, no action or opinion was deemed necessary by the D.O.'s at that time.[6]

In February, 1944, the COA committee was advised by its counterpart that both the council and the American Association of Medical Colleges had given their tentative approval. However, within a month the Federation of State Medical Boards announced it would refuse to recognize the validity of such an M.D. degree, and warned that any college issuing it would lose the right to have any of its regular graduates examined for licensure. Furthermore, strong oppostion was also voiced by certain influential AMA leaders, notably Morris Fishbein, M.D., editor of *JAMA,* who was ready to fight any accommodation between "physicians" and "cultists."[7] These moves in turn forced the American Association of Medical Colleges and the council to back away from their previous stance. At the Spring 1944 COA convention, the head of the Fact-Finding Committee noted that any possibility for amalgamation in the near future had disappeared.[8]

The central AOA headquarters staff in Chicago and key national leaders around the country were kept apprised through their local contacts of the events in California. Their strategy seems to have been to do and say nothing. First, they did not want to be viewed as interfering in that state's association affairs; if they were to do so, those who favored a merger might capitalize upon the issue and gain support. Second, they believed that the merger talk was just that. And third, they believed this effort to be triggered by the desire to obtain an M.D. degree just to be eligible to serve in the military medical corps. Once victory overseas had been achieved, sentiment in this direction would undoubtedly pass. As a result of the AOA's decision not to print any information or commentary in its journals, the great majority of D.O.'s outside California remained ignorant of the entire matter.

In the late 1940s, however, the attention of the profession was focused upon that state when a group of dissident D.O.'s set up their own "medical college" for the purpose of granting "academic" M.D. degrees to any osteopathic physician and surgeon who paid his tuition fee and attended thirty-six hours of lectures. During 1947 and 1948, at least 137 D.O.'s secured one of these M.D. degrees. Graduates of this institution, known as Metropolitan University, then set up what was called the Pacific Medical Association, which began lobbying for its own legislative program.[9]

Both the COA and the AOA took a strong stand against these activities. In 1948 the AOA house unanimously amended the code of ethics to prevent any D.O. from possessing or displaying any unaccredited degree, and through national and COA pressure, both the Metropolitan University and the Pacific Medical Association were forced to disband the following year.[10] The position taken by the COA in this matter seemed to convince many of those AOA leaders acquainted with the merger attempt a few years earlier that such a threat had in fact passed. However, the action of the COA was primarily motivated by its belief that the Metropolitan people with their worthless degrees were embarrassing the profession and that the establishment of a rival lobbying group would only sap its own political strength. Indeed, the desire for a merger by many COA leaders and the membership had not diminished, and informal discussions with the CMA on how this goal might be achieved continued, unbeknownst to the AOA.[11]

Both D.O. and M.D. discussants in these continuing COA-CMA talks came to recognize that as long as the medical profession generally and AMA officials in particular held a decidedly negative view of osteopathy, a merger would be most difficult, if not impossible, to arrange. One possible way to break down this hostility would be to get their respective national leaders to hold conferences about common concerns. Such interactions could very well lead to a better understanding between the two larger associations and an upgrading of the status of the D.O.'s, which in turn would facilitate their local efforts.[12]

In 1949 the COA House of Delegates, through its representatives, urged the AOA Board of Trustees to establish a fact-finding committee that would be prepared to meet with "any group of the healing arts." The Californians argued that in recent years its own Fact-Finding Committee had been able to resolve differences with the CMA as well as with other state health associations over proposed legislation, and reduce mutual mistrust. If any of the AOA board members were skeptical as to the motivation behind the California proposal, they kept their doubts off the public record. Instead, the board quickly and quietly approved the measure, although the mechanics of how such talks might be initiated, particularly with the AMA, remained unresolved for more than a year.[13]

In October, 1950, Floyd Peckham, D.O. of New York, president-elect of the AOA, addressed the Kentucky Osteopathic Association. At the instigation of a D.O. member of the state board of health, he was able to meet informally with AMA president Elmer Henderson, a local resident. During their friendly chat, the legal problem faced by the Chicago College of Osteopathy was raised. Although its graduates were then eligible in thirty-five states for unlimited licensure, this was not true in Illinois itself. As a result of their talk, both agreed that a conference should be arranged between representatives of their associations to discuss this matter in greater depth.[14] In December the AOA board appointed a five-man committee that included two Californians, which met with a similar group from the AMA in February, 1951. At this meeting the M.D.'s were of one mind that the question of the Chicago school was a matter for local, not national, action, and so with the D.O.'s acquiescence, the matter was dropped. Some of the M.D.'s in turn brought up the issue of amalgamation of the two professions, but this was coldly received. In all, nothing of substance was accomplished, yet despite this lack of agreement on topics for discussion, it was the feeling of the participants that future conferences might prove useful.[15]

That June, newly installed AMA president and Conference Committee member John W. Cline, M.D. of California, reported to his Board of Trustees that "the relations between medicine and osteopathy present . . . widespread problems involving a majority of the states to some degree," and he therefore urged that it appoint a committee for the second time to discuss these matters with AOA representatives.[16] The board acceded to this request and soon afterwards a similar committee was appointed by the AOA. At this conference, held in March, 1952, discussion centered on the question of the longstanding AMA position designating the D.O.'s as "cultists." This, all parties agreed, was an obvious stumbling block to overcome if the two associations were to resolve other problems, particularly the matter of interprofessional consultation between practitioners and the issue of D.O.'s and M.D.'s being on the staffs of public hospitals. This meeting ended with a greater degree of understanding on both sides.[17]

In his farewell presidential speech in June, 1952, Dr. Cline, addressing the AMA House of Delegates, briefly mentioned the work of the Conference Committee, declaring that osteopathy had in recent years come much closer to medicine and that "removal of the stigma of cultism would hasten that process." As a first step, Cline recommended that the Council on Medical Education and Hospitals be permitted to aid and advise osteopathic schools, and that any ethical barrier now preventing M.D.'s from teaching in these colleges be removed. No action was taken on Cline's suggestions, though the board agreed to let its Conference Committee meet again with the AOA "when or if requested." Meanwhile, the Judicial Council was asked to prepare an opinion.[18]

Up until this time, the Conference Committee discussions had taken place without the knowledge of the rank and file of either profession. However, with Cline's address the meetings had become public. In some osteopathic circles this news was interpreted as meaning that the two associations were conspiring to arrange a merger, which in turn caused an outpouring of angry letters, telegrams, and phone calls to AOA headquarters from outraged D.O.'s in the field. In successfully allaying their fears, the AOA board and house in July, 1952, reaffirmed "in the strongest terms possible the policy of maintaining a separate, complete and distinctive school of medicine." This was followed up by editorials in AOA publications explaining the history of the Conference Committees and the content of the discussions to date.[19]

In December, 1953, the AMA House of Delegates was informed by the Judicial Council that it had no report from the Conference Committee that had been appointed in June. Lacking any additional information on osteopathy, it could do nothing more than "reassert its opinion that all voluntary associations with osteopaths are unethical." Cline, who had been made head of the committee, pointed out in response that the wording of the June resolution, namely that they would meet "when or if requested," was holding up future talks. As a result, the AMA removed the troublesome precondition, giving Cline a free hand. The AOA board in response gave its committee a similar charge, and another meeting was scheduled.[20]

In preparation for this third session, Cline set about collecting what historical and current data on osteopathy—its schools, hospitals, laws—he could find. He and other committee members consulted with various D.O.'s and the AOA central office staff, and sent out questionnaires to osteopathic colleges as to the elements of osteopathic education. When the two conference committees met in May, 1953, they jointly reviewed the information the M.D.'s had gathered, with the AOA representatives furnishing new materials.[21]

The following month Cline presented a detailed report to the AMA Board of Trustees on osteopathy for their consideration. In it he noted that while the original teachings of Andrew Taylor Still "could be classified as 'cultist' healing," a great evolutionary change had since taken place within the profession. While he was unable historically to trace this progress due to an absence of adequate secondary sources, Cline observed that over the past several decades osteopathic colleges had fully integrated pharmacology, surgery, and all other orthodox modalities into their curriculum and had reduced the time allocated to distinctively osteopathic features. Furthermore, the "osteopathic concept" or philosophy had been broadened. Though D.O.'s had differences of opinion among themselves in this regard, the concept consisted of three basic principles: first, the normal body contains within itself the mechanisms of defense and repair in injuries resulting from trauma, infections, and other toxic agents; second, the body is a unit, and abnormal structure or function in one part exerts abnormal influence in other parts; and third, the body can function best in defense and repair when it is in correct structural alignment. Cline went on to describe the colleges in terms of their facilities, class sizes, curriculum, and quality of instruction. He noted the geographic distribution of D.O.'s, the volume of care they delivered, the scope of licensure, postgraduate education, and the current state of relationships between M.D.'s and D.O.'s. In concluding his presentation, Cline and his committee made four recommendations: (1) that the House of Delegates declare that so little of the original concept of osteopathy remained it does not classify medicine as currently taught in osteopathic schools as the teaching of cultist healing; (2) that it be the policy of the association to encourage improvement in undergraduate and postgraduate education of doctors of osteopathy; (3) that the state medical associations determine for themselves whether professional relations between M.D.'s and D.O.'s were ethical; and (4) that the Conference Committee be established on a continuous basis. After mulling the matter over, the AMA board decided because of the length of the report and the controversial nature of the subject that the House of Delegates would need further time for its study and, in addition, that the state associations should have the opportunity to express their opinions. The committee was continued, but action on the report was deferred for one year until June, 1954.[22]

The following September, Floyd Peckham, D.O., head of the AOA Conference Committee, telephoned Cline to express appreciation for his efforts and find out if there was anything more he could do to assist him in removing the cultist label. Cline, in response, suggested the possibility of on-campus visits by his committee of osteopathic schools, explaining that the most telling criticism of his report was that his information was secondhand and hearsay. While he himself knew the data to be reliable and his statements factual, this did not satisfy the skeptics, and many of these individuals would have to be won over if his recommendations were to have a chance of passage next year. An on-campus visit by the committee, accompanied by distinguished medical educators, would help to undermine the opposition.[23]

In October the AOA Conference Committee formally met and Peckham conveyed the substance of his conversation with Cline. The committee agreed that they would give his plan due consideration when it was submitted, but that this was a matter to be decided by the Board of Trustees. Early in December, following the annual AMA house meetings, Cline telephoned Peckham with the news that he had cleared his proposal with all the necessary authorities within the AMA and now had the power to relay to him the details of his plan, which he did in a letter dated December 8, 1953. Cline suggested the same type of unfocused, comprehensive survey carried out by the Council on Medical Education and Hospitals for the purposes of accreditation. Peckham immediately realized that this would be unacceptable; nevertheless, a special session of the AOA board was convened for a hearing. As expected, the Cline proposal was formally rejected; however, the board decided not to preclude the possibility of any on-site visitations per se. It instead directed its Conference Committee to meet with its counterpart to see if they could agree on a satisfactory compromise.[24]

On January 16, 1954, the two conference committees again met, whereupon the D.O.'s listed a number of conditions they believed would facilitate approval of a visitation; first, a passage within the AMA proposal stating clearly that their on-campus inspection would have nothing to do with accreditation and affirming that the AOA Bureau of Professional Education and Colleges was the only authoritative body that had the right to accredit osteopathic schools, and that under no circumstances was it the will of that committee to disturb or upset that responsibility; second, wording to the effect that the primary purpose of the visitation was to determine whether or not "medicine as currently taught in schools of osteopathy constitutes the teaching of 'cultist healing'"; and third, the establishment of the right of the

AOA to reject any of the visitation advisors proposed by the AMA. Cline and his committee immediately accepted all of these conditions.[25]

The following month another special meeting of the AOA board was convened which was attended by a representative from each osteopathic college, as well as by other key members of the profession. Cline's revised proposal, despite integrating all of the suggestions made by Peckham's committee, still met with serious objections. Some board members were afraid that the resulting report would be negative and therefore might seriously harm the profession in its legislative efforts. They had not forgotten the problems caused by the Etherington-Ryerson survey of some two decades earlier. Also, there was the fear of the outcome should the report be favorable. This might signify to lawmakers that the need for independent boards had passed and in this way give impetus to the push for their elimination. Furthermore, a positive report might lead the AMA not only to remove the cultist label, but to launch a campaign to bring about complete amalgamation. These doubts led the board to defer immediate action and to put the matter before the next regular session of the House of Delegates, which was to meet one month after Cline's original recommendations were to be voted upon.[26]

At the AMA board and house meetings in June, Cline won approval of another year's delay based on the prospect of an AMA inspection of osteopathic schools in fact taking place. This left the decision to the D.O.'s. During its sessions in July, the AOA house debated the same issues that had come up at the February board meeting. This time, however, the members of the Conference Committee took a far more active role in the discussion, arguing that unless the AMA visitation was approved, there was no chance that the cultist label would be removed. This proved decisive. The opposition was overcome and the Conference Committee was given full authority to negotiate with its counterpart in making final arrangements.[27]

### The AMA Inspection

Under the terms of the agreement between the two associations, each osteopathic school had the right to decide whether or not it would participate in the inspections. By late October, all the colleges except one had given their approval; the Philadelphia school argued that the visitation still looked too much like an accreditation process and therefore declined. As the original AMA mandate called for a survey of all the colleges, Cline's committee had to wait until the AMA clinical meeting in December to receive official authorization to inspect only five.[28]

Prior to visitation, which took place between January and March, 1955, each school filled out a questionnaire patterned after that required of colleges seeking accreditation by the Council on Medical Education and Hospitals to provide essential information concerning organization, authority, administration, finances, facilities, and operation of the colleges; the personnel, training, authority, and activities of the faculty; the curriculum content; the organization of departments, their objectives, methods of teaching, and equipment; the degree of interdepartmental coordination and cooperation; and the details of library facilities and contents.

Each institution was visited by at least two members of the committee, which then consisted of John Cline, M.D., James Z. Appel, M.D., Leonard Larson, M.D., Thomas P. Murdock, M.D., and Cleon A. Nafe, M.D., accompanied by one of the mutually agreed upon educational advisors: L. R. Chandler, M.D., recently retired dean of the Stanford University School of Medicine, J. Murray Kinsman, M.D., dean of the University of Louisville School of Medicine, and W. Clarke Wescoe, M.D., dean of the University of Kansas School of Medicine. The committee team of each school was accompanied by Floyd F. Peckham, D.O., AOA Conference Committee chairman.

It was agreed beforehand that the inspection committee would have access to all the information they believed essential to their efforts and that the observations would be of such breadth, depth, and duration as they deemed necessary. At the end of each on-site visit, the advisor prepared a report, one copy of which was transmitted to the college, while the other was held by the AMA committee as a confidential document.

Following completion of all visitations, the committee drafted a final document containing the answers to four questions posed to it by the AMA board: (1) Is modern osteopathic education the teaching of "cultist" medicine within the definition of the principles of medical ethics? (2) If the first question is at all true, to what degree? (3) If to some degree, does this element interfere with sound medical education? and (4) What is the quality of medical education?

In its findings, presented to the AMA House of Delegates in June, 1955, the committee noted that all of the schools were attempting to give their students a rounded general practitioner type of training, expecting that the majority of their graduates would become primary care physicians and that a high percentage would locate in traditionally underserved communities. Examining student records, the committee observed that all students had completed the educational requirements for admission to an AMA-accredited college and that a considerable number of them could have obtained admission to medical school. Interviews conducted with students revealed that the motivation to become physicians was strong in most. While some were disappointed medical school applicants, more had previous contacts with the osteopathic profession and were thereby influenced to enter D.O.

schools. A small number, in fact, had been accepted by M.D. colleges but chose osteopathy instead.

All the schools, the committee observed, were handicapped by limited finances; endowments were small or nonexistent, and too much of their funding was derived from tuition. At one institution, student fees accounted for more than 50 percent of the total income. Because of this inadequate financial situation, the schools were not able to hire more full-time faculty and improve their facilities and equipment to the extent that the colleges would have liked. Though the committee noted that in recent years additional sources of funding (for example, the Osteopathic Progress Fund; federal teaching grants; and Hill-Burton monies) had allowed the schools to make some significant progress, considerably more support was necessary.

In terms of curriculum, the committe found that the clock hours of osteopathic instruction exceeded those of schools of medicine by several hundred. This, it felt, was not advantageous to the student since it crowded too much into too limited a period. As a result, there was little time for individual student projects, library use, and reflection and assimilation of the knowledge the student acquired. Furthermore, the situation did not encourage a scholarly attitude or an interest in research.

In the basic sciences, it concluded that the subjects were fairly well taught and that the students were well grounded in these fields. Some departments —most frequently anatomy—were outstanding, although some, particularly pathology, were comparatively poor due to a shortage of trained personnel. In the clinical years, the committee believed that there was too much didactic teaching and a tendency to treat the student as an observer rather than as a part of the patient care team. The methods and quality of clinical instruction, it found, varied from school to school, and to a considerable degree in different courses within the same college. A similar finding was made of the qualifications, teaching abilities, and interests of the faculty members. Finally, the committee felt that the clinical material available was inadequate for the number of students in a majority of the colleges.

On the most controversial aspects of osteopathic instruction, the committee believed that what was being taught simply reflected a difference in both theory and practice emphases between M.D.'s and D.O.'s, rather than a conflict between science and nonscience. What D.O.'s referred to as the "osteopathic concept" was merely the expression of these differences. "Modern osteopathic education," its report noted, "teaches the acceptance and recognition of all etiological factors and all pathological manifestations of disease as well as the utilization of all diagnostic and therapeutic procedures taught in schools of medicine."[29]

In the committee's view, osteopathic manipulation had been relegated to the status of an adjunct to therapy within the sphere of medicine. Nowhere did it find it to occupy a preeminent place in instruction. When applied to hospital inpatients with clinically recognized disease, for example, it found it consisted mainly of relaxing, soft tissue manipulation or that designed to increase respiratory excursion. Some heads of clinical departments believed it had considerable value in conjunction with standard therapy while others did not. "The use of manipulative therapy," it observed, "is decreasing in colleges of osteopathy and is increasing in the orthopedic and physiology departments of medical schools."[30]

At the conclusion of its report the committee restated, though in somewhat revised form, the recommendations originally submitted in 1953. It urged the house to declare that current education in osteopathic colleges did not constitute the teaching of cultist healing; that M.D.'s be encouraged to assist in osteopathic pre- and postgraduate training programs in those states where such participation is not contrary to the announced policy of the state medical association; that these same state associations assume the responsibility of determining the ethical relationship between M.D.'s and D.O.'s, or request their component county societies to do so; and that the Conference Committee be continued to meet with AOA representatives concerning common or interprofessional problems at the national level.[31]

Upon submission, the report was sent to the AMA Reference Committee on Medical Education and Hospitals, which in turn presented a majority and minority opinion. Both declared that, unlike the inspection team, they were not satisfied that current education in D.O. schools was free of the teaching of "cultist healing." However, beyond this the two sharply differed. The majority report, representing four out of the five members of the Reference Committee, urged the passage of the Conference Committee's last three recommendations. The minority report, consisting of the views of one member, Milford O. Rouse, M.D. of Texas, urged rejection of all four recommendations and the adoption of two substitutes; first, that the Conference Committee be thanked for its diligent work and be discontinued, and second, "that if and when the House of Delegates of the American Osteopathic Association, its official policy-making body, may voluntarily abandon the commonly so called 'osteopathic concept,' with proper deletion of said 'osteopathic concept' from catalogs of their colleges and may approach the Board of Trustees of the American Medical Association with a request for further discussion of the relations of osteopathy and medicine, then the said Trustees shall appoint another special committee for such discussion." After a vigorous and emotional debate on the floor of the house, the motion to adopt the majority report was amended to substitute the minority report in its place. Upon further discussion, the house by a vote of 101 to 81 passed the Rouse resolutions. All the findings of the college inspection team were thus repudiated, and the D.O.'s officially remained "cultists" in the eyes of the AMA.[32]

## An Amalgamation in California

The reaction of the AOA Conference Committee members who met two days after the AMA house vote was one of bitter disappointment. Although they were far from pleased with the Cline Report in its entirety they concluded that on the whole it was reasonably fair. As far as the decision of the AMA house was concerned, it simply reinforced their belief that politics was at the heart of the cultism issue.[33] At the AOA House of Delegates meeting the following month, the actions of the AMA were largely ignored in the official sessions. The association restated its position of cooperation with any group whenever such cooperation may be expected to lead to the improved health service of the American people. It retained its national Conference Committee for that purpose and urged the establishment of similar committees on the local level.[34]

As in the case of their national association, leaders of the California Osteopathic Association were greatly upset by the AMA house vote on the Cline Report. Nevertheless, they clearly recognized that the on-site visitations had opened many of the delegates' eyes as to what was actually taught in osteopathic schools, and in so doing helped to raise their standing and status among M.D.'s generally. What now remained to be done to facilitate a local merger was to push the AOA towards meeting the Rouse conditions, so that the stigma of the cultist label would be removed, thereby eliminating any possible AMA objections to amalgamation. At its May, 1957, meeting, the COA House of Delegates passed a resolution urging the deletion from all AOA printed materials those statements referring to the osteopathic profession as a separate, independent, and complete school of therapy, and the removal of all possibly "cultist" terminology employed by the colleges and hospitals, and directed its delegation to the AOA house to make every effort to implement these changes.[35]

That July, during the national convention, debate centered on the AOA constitution, which then read in part:

> The objects of this Association shall be to promote the public health and the art and science of the osteopathic school of practice of the healing art, by maintaining high standards of osteopathic education and by advancing the profession's knowledge of surgery, obstetrics, and the prevention, diagnosis and treatment of disease in general; by stimulating original research and investigation, and by collecting and disseminating the results of such work for the education and improvement of the profession and the ultimate benefit of humanity; that the evolution of the osteopathic principles shall be an ever growing tribute to Andrew Taylor Still whose original researches made possible osteopathy as a science.[36]

In place of this awkward, "cultist"-sounding testament, a majority of the members of a Special Reference Committee of the house proposed that this part of the constitution, known as article 2, be amended to read "The objects of this Association shall be to promote the public health to encourage scientific research and to improve high standards of medical education." This was moved by California on the house floor. A minority report, supported by Michigan representatives, strongly argued that this statement led to questionable interpretations and urged substitution of the term *osteopathic education* for *medical education*. A seemingly certain and bitter floor fight between the two largest delegations was narrowly averted when both sides agreed to compromise language: *medical education in osteopathic colleges*. This change was thus approved for publication and set for final action at the next year's meeting, where the house overwhelmingly approved it.[37]

At the December, 1958, meeting of the AMA house, the Indiana delegation, following the Cline recommendations, again proposed that the state societies be given the responsibility for determining whether relations between M.D.'s and D.O.'s were ethical. This was rejected once more; however, the committee studying this resolution made the suggestion, which was approved, that the Judicial Council consider this matter further and submit a report.[38] During the next house meeting in June, 1959, the Judicial Council, specifically citing the recent AOA constitutional changes, now proposed a significant revision of association policy, recommending, "It shall not be considered contrary to the Principles of Medical Ethics for members of the A.M.A. voluntarily to associate professionally with physicians other than doctors of medicine, who are licensed to practice the healing art without restriction and who base their practice on the same scientific principles as those adhered to by members of the A.M.A. [and for A.M.A. members] to teach students of osteopathic medicine who seek to develop and improve their ability to provide a better quality of medical care."[39]

To the surprise of many, this was opposed by the California delegation, which argued the changes were too generous, and which announced publically that the CMA was then actively involved in negotiations with the COA to amalgamate the two professions and take over the osteopathic college. By giving the D.O.'s all they asked for now, the bargaining position of the CMA would thus be weakened. On the AMA house floor the Californians led a successful fight amending the entire resolution to read simply, "It shall not be considered contrary to the principles of medical ethics for doctors of medicine to teach students in an osteopathic college which is in the process of being converted into an approved medical school which is under the supervision of the A.M.A. Council on Medical Education and Hospitals."[40] Needless to say, the eyes of organized osteopathy now turned towards California.

The next month at the AOA House of Delegates meeting, retiring association president George W. Northup, D.O., focused on what, apparently, was happening. In his address, Northup reviewed in some detail the discussions held in the early 1940s pertaining to merger, and noted that since then, rumors had periodically circulated that further talks along these lines were being held. Now with the public statement by CMA representatives that a merger between the two California groups was imminent, some clear and straightforward answers were due the AOA by its divisional society. Northup forcefully stated:

> In fairness to the remainder of the profession, its educational system, and its programs for the future, this profession and the House of Delegates has the right, yes, the responsibility to know whether there is any validity in these statements so that the AOA can act accordingly. If we are about to lose one of our prominent and best qualified colleges, we should face the possibility fairly and honestly. If the largest divisional organization of this profession is conducting through its leadership, official or unofficial, private negotiations with one of the largest divisional medical societies which might lead to the loss of their membership in the AOA that too must be faced realistically and honestly.

Northup then asked the House of Delegates four questions:

> (1) Do we wish to maintain the independence of our colleges or do we desire to convert them into medical schools under the supervision and jurisdiction of the Council on Medical Education and Hospitals of the A.M.A.?, (2) Do we wish to take steps leading to the abandonment of our intern and residency training programs, our approved and registered hospitals; our certification and recognition of our specialists and their certifying programs; our program of development and recognition of our general practitioners; and our hard earned acceptance of the A.O.A. as a recognized accrediting agency, or are all of these to be turned over and placed under the protective custody of agencies of the A.M.A.?, (3) Do we or do we not have a contribution to make to medicine not now being accomplished through the efforts of any other organization?, (4) Do we wish to continue as an independent osteopathic profession, cooperative with all and subservient to none?[41]

Each of Northup's questions seemingly was answered with demonstrations of loyalty from all present except the California delegation, which sat stunned, angry, and silent, refusing to explain its position. Michigan's delegation then introduced a resolution in direct opposition to the California House of Delegates policy statement of 1957, reading in part, "Be it resolved that the osteopathic school of medicine, in the interest of providing the best possible health care to the public, shall maintain its status as a separate and complete school of medicine cooperating with all other agencies and groups that sincerely promote the same objective when that cooperation is on an equal basis granting full recognition to the autonomy and contribution of the osteopathic school of practice."[42] This passed ninety-five to twenty-two, with California providing the nays.

Despite this action, secret negotiations between leaders of the COA and the CMA continued apace.[43] When in early 1960 word of these talks filtered back to AOA officials, a full accounting was demanded. At the July, 1960, AOA house meeting the Californians asked for and received permission to present their case before a closed-door executive session. Drs. Dorothy Marsh and Nicholas Oddo reviewed past differences with the AOA over legislation and setting of standards, noted the problems of obtaining adequate postgraduate training, observed the inadequate financing of all phases of osteopathic education, the poor status of the D.O. degree, as well as the D.O.'s' exclusion from group health insurance plans. The profession, they maintained, was simply not moving fast enough to resolve these problems. Through amalgamation, these difficulties could be eliminated.[44] D.O.'s opposed to merger, while acknowledging the enumerated problems, argued that they could be successfully dealt with in other ways. The Californians simply wanted a quick fix, and in the process they were willing to sell out their heritage. On returning to open session, the house resolved: "That any divisional society which is in the process of negotiation leading to unification and/or 'amalgamation' or merger, or a process of a similar nature, of the osteopathic profession with or into any other organized profession involved in health care shall cease such negotiations or be subject to the revocation of its charter by the A.O.A."[45]

Now for the first time under a direct threat, the COA leadership notified its members that it was instructing its Fact-Finding Committee to cease its discussion with the CMA. However, on November 13 the full COA house, in a defiant mood, voted sixty-six to forty to ignore the AOA directive and resume talks. The AOA board reacted quickly. Meeting in special session the following week, it voted eighteen to one to revoke the COA charter.[46] This left the COA in a precarious position, particularly if a merger agreement could not be worked out. In early December a new group known as the Osteopathic Physicians and Surgeons of California (OPSC) was organized and quickly chartered as the official AOA divisional society.[47] Hopes by the OPSC leadership that it would soon represent over half the D.O.'s in the state soon proved unrealistic, however, as it was only able to attract about one-sixth of all California D.O.'s to its ranks. As Kisch and Viseltear observed, the AOA decision to remove the COA charter had the unanticipated effect of increasing the COA's social solidarity.[48]

By May, 1961, a contract between the CMA and COA was ready to be acted upon by each House of Delegates. The executive vice-president of the AMA had already assured the CMA that if unification was effected, "it would not be reviewed by any board or agency of the AMA for the purpose of approving or disapproving it."[49] This was essential, for the cultist label had not been removed and it was quite possible that the AMA house, if it had the chance, might very well veto the merger plan. Among the major provisions of the contract were, first, that the College of Osteopathic Physicians and Surgeons (COP&S), which would change its name to the California College of Medicine, would offer to all of its living graduates and those D.O.'s from other schools who held valid physician and surgeon licenses in the state a Doctor of Medicine (M.D.) degree. This would be an academic degree, the recognition of which for the purposes of licensure would depend upon the laws of the various states. However, in California, statutory provision would be made to accept it for all purposes connected with the practice of medicine. Second, those D.O.'s who chose to accept this M.D. degree would thereafter cease to identify themselves as osteopathic practitioners in any manner. Third, the California College of Medicine (formerly COP&S) would henceforth be a medical school affiliated with the Association of American Medical Colleges and end its teaching of osteopathy. Fourth, the CMA would absorb ex-D.O.'s within the existing forty-county medical society structure, although during the transition period they would be segregated into a special forty-first society. Finally, the ex-D.O.'s would support legislative action implementing the agreement, including the revision of the 1922 osteopathic initiative that gave them an independent board, to insure there would be no new future licensing of D.O.'s in the state. Those D.O.'s already licensed in California who decided not to join the merger would still come under the jurisdiction of the osteopathic board until they numbered fewer than forty, in which case it would be completely abolished and its activities taken over by the M.D. board.[50]

On May 3 the CMA house passed the agreement by a vote of 296 to 63. Two weeks later the COA house voted 100 to 10 to accept it. Later that month the Board of Trustees of COP&S, assured by representatives of inspectors from the Association of American Medical Colleges that with some relatively minor organizational and staffing changes their institution would become a fully accredited medical school, narrowly voted 13 to 11 to go along with conversion. On the fourteenth and fifteenth of July, some two thousand D.O.'s, meeting in the auditorium of Los Angeles County General Hospital, received their new M.D. degrees.[51]

After these actions the battle over the osteopathic initiative, played out the next year, seemed anticlimactic. This measure was supported by the ex-D.O.'s, the CMA, both houses of the legislature, the Democratic governor, Pat Brown, and his Republican challenger, Richard Nixon, as well as numerous civic organizations. The OPSC, which had been unable to stop any of the previous legal steps on the road to amalgamation through the courts, had to face this opposition alone. A pledge by the AOA to provide a sizable war chest had to be withdrawn when it became obvious that such a political contribution would remove the association's tax-exempt standing, since it, unlike the AMA, was registered as an educational organization with the Internal Revenue Service. With OPSC unable to generate sufficient capital to get its message across, defeat was all but assured. A final count of the votes revealed 3,407,957, or 69 percent, marking their ballots "yes"; only 1,536,470, or 31 percent, registered "no." The merger had been completed.[52]

# CHAPTER NINE

# *Reaffirmation and Expansion*

To many outside observers the events taking place in California, from the initial public announcement of a merger plan to its implementation in 1962, seemed to signal the first step in the inevitable absorption of the D.O.'s as a group into the regular medical profession. Whatever agreements had to be worked out, and however long it took, complete countrywide amalgamation was viewed as a foregone conclusion. There was no possibility that the M.D.'s would continue to let the D.O.'s remain independent or that the AOA could continue to resist the pull of the AMA upon its members. Movements such as osteopathy, homeopathy, and eclecticism, it was generally believed, have a natural life cycle. They are conceived by a crisis in medical care; their youth is marked by a broadening of their ideas; and their decline occurs when whatever distinctive notions they have as to patient management are allowed to wither. At this point, no longer having a compelling raison d'être, they die. While examples of this pattern are not difficult to find in the United States and elsewhere, this type of explanation tends to downplay, if not ignore, specific highly individualized historical conditions. Whether osteopathy would be able to survive the California merger intact or would go the way of homeopathy and eclecticism would not depend upon some deductively arrived at natural law, but upon actual social circumstances over time.

### California Aftermath

Throughout the 1950s it was readily apparent that the AMA could not forge any coherent national policy with respect to the D.O.'s. Indeed, if the AMA executive secretary had not ruled that the amalgamation being arranged in California was a local matter and therefore not subject to action by the House of Delegates, it is entirely possible that the final agreement would not have been allowed. In succeeding years this lack of uniformity and consistency on the part of the AMA as well as other significant groupings within organized medicine would severely hamper their efforts to obtain what, for them, would be a satisfactory conclusion to the osteopathic issue.

In June, 1961, while the California merger was still in process, the AMA Judicial Council delivered a special report on the association's position with respect to voluntary relations between M.D.'s and D.O.'s. Noting that "there cannot be two distinct sources of medicine or two different yet equally valid systems of medical practice," it declared that the changes occurring within osteopathy indicated the desire by a significant number of D.O.'s to give their patients scientific medical care. Because of this, "Policy should now be applied individually at [the] local level according to the facts as they exist. The test should now be: Does the individual doctor of osteopathy practice osteopathy or does he in fact practice a method of healing founded on the scientific basis? If he practices osteopathy, he practices a cult system of healing, and all voluntary professional associations with him are unethical. If he bases his practice on the same scientific principles as those adhered to by members of the American Medical Association, voluntary professional relations with him should be deemed ethical."[1]

Many AMA house delegates thought this proposed policy was far too liberal, since it would serve to make the issue of ethical relations subject to the individual M.D.'s discretion. A number of component societies, particularly those whose states restricted practice rights for D.O.'s, continued to be bitterly opposed to any interprofessional contact and thus were unwilling to support the report as it stood. As a compromise, it was amended to give each state society the right to make the determination as to whether or not its members could voluntarily associate with osteopathic practitioners on a professional basis. In this form, with almost the exact wording of the 1955 Cline committee recommendation, the policy was approved.[2] The Judicial Council also urged that local liaison committees, if not already in existence, should be established to conduct talks with their D.O. counterparts, and this was fully accepted. In some states, its report noted, "It might be possible to initiate and complete negotiations such as have been and are being carried out in California."[3] To assist the state societies in the formulation and carrying out of their plans, the AMA board created the Committee on Osteopathy and Medicine the following year.

While the AMA was characterized by sharp division within its official ranks over the question of M.D.-D.O. relations, the AOA was for its part united, both at the national and state levels. At its July, 1961, annual meeting held in Chicago, the AOA delegates in strong language reaffirmed the so-called "Michigan Resolution" of 1959 which declared their intent to maintain the status of osteopathy as a separate and complete school of medicine. Coupled with this was a sharply worded statement by the AOA board attacking the premises of the Judicial Council report. It noted:

It may be true that there cannot be two sciences of medicine, but the A.M.A. fails to recognize that while medicine employs scientific knowledge, the *practice* of medicine is not science per se. It is unrealistic to hold that the practice of medicine is pure science. It is equally unrealistic to insist that only one system of medical practice, that system officially approved by a political body, can be valid. . . . The A.M.A. holds that if an individual doctor of osteopathy practices osteopathy he is a cultist and all voluntary professional associations with him are unethical. However, if he bases his practice on the same scientific principles as those adhered to by members of the A.M.A. voluntary relationships are ethical. This policy has two fallacies: First, it assumes that the osteopathic concepts are diametrically opposed to accepted scientific fact and that osteopathic physicians do not employ accepted scientific principles in their practice. Second, it condemns a system of practice without understanding or defining it, or, in fact, defining what *is* accepted scientific medical practice.[4]

As for the mechanisms of declaring whether relations between M.D.'s and D.O.'s were ethical, the house stated that by granting their state societies the right to decide who shall and shall not be legitimate, the AMA hoped that the profession would be weakened from within and that through internal dissension it would ultimately be eliminated. "The osteopathic profession," it declared, "will continue as a separate and complete school of medical practice and . . . it will resist all efforts to be absorbed, amalgamated or destroyed, be it through overt political maneuvering, or through the guise of making its individual members conform to the scientific dictates of the A.M.A."[5]

In dealing with liaison committees established by state medical associations, the AOA divisional societies adopted a common strategy. When approached, the osteopathic representatives would announce that before any other interprofessional matter could be brought up, all medical society restrictions on voluntary M.D.-D.O. relations had to be removed. In those cases where this was done, the D.O.'s then agreed to discuss mutual problems, though they turned a deaf ear to the subject of amalgamation. As a result, by 1965 only fourteen state medical associations had approved voluntary interprofessional relations. In some states the M.D.'s held this issue hostage to merger negotiations; in others, M.D. antipathy towards the D.O.'s precluded any formal discussions whatsoever.[6]

While organized osteopathy was united against amalgamation, there was some dissension within the rank and file. However, unlike California, where absorption proponents were an active force within their state society and controlled political offices, and were thus able to maneuver the COA towards their desired goal, in other states D.O.'s who supported the merger concept were more likely not to be members of the AOA or their divisional society; and if they were members, they had not attained positions of influence. Opposition to the AOA policy line, therefore, was mostly scattered, unorganized, and lacking in effective leadership. The one exception occurred in the state of Washington, where in 1962 a faction of dissident D.O.'s broke away from the official state osteopathic association, formed their own group, and sought to arrange a merger between themselves and the state medical society. With the support of the latter, they founded a "paper college" to award M.D. degrees valid for the purposes of licensure to "qualified" Washington D.O.'s. Nothing came of this, however, as the state supreme court, in a unanimous ruling, declared that the Board of Medical Examiners' decision to approve the paper college as a medical school was "subterfuge, was palpably arbitrary and capricious, and was void in all respects."[7]

A significant number of D.O.'s around the country were simply undecided about merger. Troubled by their own special problems, whether it be poor public perception, denial of staff privileges at local hospitals, or ineligibility for participation in prepaid insurance plans, they harbored genuine doubts as to the wisest position for them to take. To help counter such wavering, the AOA organized and conducted a series of "regional town meetings" across the country in which officials explained recently adopted policy positions as well as the association's efforts on the legislative and judicial fronts to break down discriminatory barriers.[8] While such gatherings in which the fears and frustrations of concerned D.O.'s were openly aired and seriously addressed by AOA leaders served to convince some who attended of the "rightness" of the association's stand, other D.O.'s adopted a wait-and-see attitude, letting time pass to enable them to determine for themselves how well the California plan was working out before coming to any hard-and-fast conclusions.

In the years following the California merger it became evident to the ex-D.O.'s who participated that their move had both positive and negative features. On the favorable side, the vast majority seemed to be quite happy with the new M.D. initials behind their name. Although one AOA leader warned them that they and members of their family would be forever subjected to the whisper, "He is an osteopath who was given an M.D. degree," this did not appear to be a significant problem.[9] Patients readily accepted the changed designation as well as the new diploma on the wall, and most ex-D.O.'s felt relieved at no longer having to answer such questions as, "What kind of doctor are you anyway?"[10]

The most satisfied of the ex-D.O.'s were clearly the general practitioners. Aside from their new degrees, they found they could now obtain admitting privileges at hospitals that had once barred them, that their malpractice rates as a result of joining the CMA were substantially lower than they had been previously, and that they could freely consult with a wider range of specialists.[11]

Nevertheless, major problems did surface. As part of the amalgamation contract, all ex-D.O.'s were to be temporarily segregated in a special forty-first component society of the CMA until they could be fully integrated into the other forty county societies. Though most of the ex-D.O.'s had no difficulty in being assimilated, a significant number did. As late as 1967, five years after amalgamation, approximately 10 percent of the original group had not been granted regular local membership. This proved to be a source of some embarrassment and discontent.[12]

Far more serious was the status of ex-D.O. specialists—a subject that was left unresolved in the merger agreement. Under the existing AMA requirements all candidates for specialty board certification had to graduate from an accredited medical school and receive his or her postgraduate training in an AMA-approved hospital program. This meant that ex-D.O.'s, including those who had been certified by an AOA board, could not receive any consideration for similar certification from its AMA counterpart. Though CMA officials reportedly pledged to work for changes in AMA policy, no movement in that direction was forthcoming. What the CMA agreed to do was to inspect the D.O. specialists' osteopathic credentials and then issue a certificate stating that they were found to be in order. While this document may have been suitable for hanging in the office to impress one's clients, it could not help the practitioner in gaining staff privileges at other than ex-osteopathic hospitals.[13] Another consequence of this lack of proper certification was a decline in the number of patients regularly referred to these specialists. Before the merger, D.O. generalists would be more likely to send a patient an inconvenient distance to see a D.O. gynecologist, internist, or surgeon. But now, as the ex-D.O. general practitioners made new professional acquaintances, they began to refer patients to specialists more on the basis of their credentials and proximity. Furthermore, most of what ex-D.O.'s in California called "congenital M.D.'s," that is, those who graduated from an AMA-accredited school, were unwilling to send patients to "acquired M.D.'s."[14]

In the years following the merger agreement, a number of ex-osteopathic hospitals found themselves in financial difficulty. Some institutions reported a staff loss of up to 20 percent, as local D.O. general practitioners began affiliating with congenital-M.D. facilities. In some cases, the loss was made up for by the addition of congenital M.D.'s to the staff, but most hospitals sampled in 1965 by the AOA reported that their occupancy rate was lower than it had been before the merger. A few institutions saw themselves as eventually going out of business or selling out, while others anticipated they would become satellite facilities for major congenital-M.D. hospitals.[15] Also, all ex-D.O. facilities lost their intern and residency programs. These institutions, with the exception of the new Los Angeles County Hospital, were simply too small to qualify for AMA approval. Thus they were no longer teaching oriented, a change not a few of the staff regreted.

What was once the College of Osteopathic Physicians and Surgeons and is now the California College of Medicine became part of the University of California state system in 1962, with a new campus being established for it at Irvine several years later. With a far greater source of revenue now at its disposal, new equipment was purchased, and many more full-time instructors were hired. As it was now an orthodox medical institution, it could become affiliated with a number of large congenital-M.D. hospitals, thus improving training opportunities. Losing out in this process were many part-time and voluntary ex-D.O. faculty members whose services were no longer required. Also affected were a number of full-time ex-D.O.'s who, while not removed from the staff, found themselves maneuvered out of positions in authority in favor of congenital M.D.'s.[16]

A final critical problem arising from the merger was the worthlessness of the acquired M.D. degree as a basis for licensure everywhere outside California. By 1966 courts in ten states had ruled in favor of those examining boards who rejected applicants from holders of the 1961 diploma on the grounds that theirs was an academic, not a professional, degree. Only those California College of Medicine students completing their training in 1962 or later were considered graduates of an AMA-accredited institution.[17]

Needless to say, the two major AOA publications, the *JAOA* and *The D.O.*, continuously pointed out and amplified all these problems to their readers as evidence that amalgamation was a failure. Editorials blasting the holders of what was labeled "the little m.d." were occasionally coupled with letters from ex-D.O.'s who voiced deep disappointment with all or certain features of the merger. Although the picture drawn by the AOA was one-sided, it was nevertheless apparent from a reading of even generally pro-merger articles in nonosteopathic journals that not everything had worked out as well as all ex-D.O.'s had hoped.[18]

These perceived inequities and difficulties only served to make many undecided D.O.'s around the country wary of amalgamation—or at least amalgamation of the California variety. In a 1972 mail survey of D.O.'s in twelve geographically scattered states conducted by the independent journal the *Osteopathic Physician,* only 17 (or 7.8 percent) of 218 practitioners responding answered "yes" to the question, "Do you view the merger in California as a satisfactory one?"[19]

In addition to the California situation, a major factor that would lead undecided D.O.'s to shy away from supporting merger was the perceived inability on the part of the AMA and other medical groups to treat them with what they believed was sufficient professional respect. Indeed, where organized medicine altered existing discriminatory policies toward the D.O.'s, its only motivation seemed to be the desire to solve the problems these policies caused for M.D.'s—not to eliminate "gross injustices" against osteopathic practitioners. For example, in 1959 the American Hospital Association decided to change its longstanding policy that barred joint or mixed staff institutions from membership only after being the subject of tremendous continuous pressure from many public hospitals that were being forced by court or legislative action to place D.O.'s on their staffs. Under its revised rules, D.O.'s could now become staff members, but general supervision of the clinical work was to remain the responsibility of M.D.'s alone.[20] American Hospital Association membership was a necessary prerequisite for eligibility for approval by the Joint Commission on the Accreditation of Hospitals, and in 1960, again only under strong pressure from the same source, the Joint Commission made the appropriate adjustments to permit these institutions to be inspected and accredited.[21] Thus, whatever victory the D.O.'s achieved in these instances was only an unavoidable byproduct of quite a different motive held by the M.D.'s.

The "true" attitude of the AMA and other medical groups could be seen in other ways. When it came to supporting opportunities and responsibilities for D.O.'s equal to those enjoyed by M.D.'s in public hospitals, organized medicine said no; when it came to changing practice laws that discriminated against D.O.'s, organized medicine was generally opposed; finally, when it came to pending federal legislation to underwrite the expenses of health profession schools, the AMA would testify that osteopathic institutions should be excluded.[22] Furthermore, many of those D.O.'s who read *JAMA* articles pertaining to osteopathy, either in the original or as reprinted elsewhere, felt denigrated or insulted by their assumptions and tone. Particularly galling was the fact that in article after article, D.O.'s were referred to as osteopaths in contradistinction to physicians—a title used to denote M.D.'s only. Based on the actions and rhetoric of the AMA, most D.O.'s seemed to have come to the conclusion that the association was not willing or perhaps incapable of dealing with them as equals. Rather, it appeared that organized medicine regarded the osteopathic profession as nothing more than a nuisance which had to be eliminated one way or another.

## The New AMA Offensive

By the mid-1960s it was apparent to the AMA leadership that organized osteopathy was standing firm. The strategy, or compromise, of letting state societies decide the cultism issue had not served to bring amalgamation closer to fruition. Furthermore, the unresolved problems of the California merger had caused considerable skepticism among individual D.O.'s. However, most distressing to the leadership had to be the fact that the merger itself was having the unintended consequence of permitting the osteopathic profession to make key political gains, thus serving to increase its strength and position.

That D.O.'s had become M.D.'s without any additional educational requirements, and especially the fact that COP&S became a fully accredited M.D.-granting institution so quickly and with comparatively few structural changes, signalled to a number of legislators in limited licensure states who were previously opposed to revising their medical practice acts that whatever gaps there might be in the quality of training between D.O.'s and M.D.'s, they were no longer significant. Thus osteopathic lobbying efforts, once at a standstill, now began to pick up considerable momentum. The merger had a similar impact on the federal level. In 1963 the United States Civil Service Commission, specifically citing events in California, announced that for its purposes the M.D. and D.O. degrees were henceforth to be considered equivalent. In 1966 Secretary of Defense Robert McNamara, using legislative authority granted to his office a decade earlier, ordered all the armed services to accept qualified D.O.'s as military physicians and surgeons for the first time. Also that same year, the AOA won a major victory when it was accepted as an accrediting agency over osteopathic hospitals for the purpose of determining an institution's eligibility for participation in the Medicare program (Public Law 89-97, July 30, 1965).[23] Thus the D.O.'s were increasingly obtaining on their own some of the benefits the M.D.'s could offer through amalgamation.

In view of these circumstances the AMA adopted a series of new resolutions in the late 1960s aimed at destroying the AOA. Designed to take away many of its colleges, students, interns, and residents, as well as a large proportion of its members, the AMA plan sought to force the issue of absorption quickly, before organized osteopathy became too powerful. The first actions came in July, 1967, when the AMA house authorized its Board of Trustees to begin negotiations promptly with all the D.O. schools for the sole purpose of converting them to orthodox medical institutions. In order to place pressure upon them to bargain, the house also authorized the Council on Medical Education "to establish means by which selected students with proven satisfactory scholastic ability in schools of osteopathy may be considered by schools of medicine for transfer into medical school classes." In short, the colleges were warned that if they resisted the AMA overture, they would soon find themselves with a sharply depleted enrollment. In adopting these actions, the house noted, "The primary issue at the present time in the relationship of medicine and osteopathy seems to be not that of cultism as opposed to science. Rather the issue appears to be one level of medical education and practice to another and lower level of medical education and practice."[24]

In response, the AOA house the following month adopted a resolution that declared in part, "The A.M.A. contention that osteopathic education needs to be improved is obviously not shared by recognized educational accrediting agencies, by state licensing bodies or by the millions of Americans who prefer osteopathic care. . . . The A.M.A. stands alone in its assessment of osteopathic education, but the osteopathic profession stands together in vigorously opposing this arrogant policy of academic piracy."[25] Indeed, the colleges did hold together, although a difficult economic situation at the Des Moines school led its administration to hold talks with AMA and Association of American Medical Colleges representatives. However, this threat to solidarity was eliminated when those college officials resigned under AOA pressure and were replaced by individuals who supported an antimerger line.[26]

Disappointed with an initial lack of movement, the AMA soon followed with two other major policy shifts. In December, 1968, the House of Delegates passed resolutions that, first, encouraged each county and state medical society to change its by-laws so that it "may accept qualified osteopaths as active members," and, second, urged that each of the boards of medical specialties change its rules in order to "accept for examination for certification those osteopaths who have completed A.M.A. approved internship and residency programs and have met the other regular requirements applicable to all board candidates." As specialty boards declared their intent to permit examination of D.O.'s, appropriate AMA-approved residency programs would be opened to qualified osteopathic graduates. Determination of qualification for acceptance into a given program would be left up to the medical staff of the hospital or to the county medical society.[27] In June, 1969, the AMA house extended to D.O.'s membership in the national association and officially changed the "Essentials of Approved Residencies," clearing the path for D.O. acceptance into those programs in which the respective specialty boards had agreed to later examine them for the purposes of certification. At that time, five boards—pathology, pediatrics, physical medicine and rehabilitation, preventitive medicine, and radiology—had done so. By 1970 the number had increased to eleven, and by 1971, thirteen.[28]

These actions posed serious potential problems for the AOA. As early as 1968 the issue of belonging to an allopathic medical association arose in connection with two D.O.'s who accepted associate membership status in the Michigan State Medical Society. The AOA house, in turn, adopted a resolution declaring that "any member accepting membership in the American Medical Association or any of its political divisions is acting contrary to the best interests of the American Osteopathic Association and shall be subject to discipline up to and including expulsion." The following July the house clarified this resolution by interpreting "political divisions" to mean national, state, divisional, or county medical societies.[29]

In 1971 both the Iowa and the Pennsylvania delegations offered resolutions to the AOA house seeking to reverse this policy. In each of these states, particularly in areas where there were no osteopathic hospitals, D.O.'s found themselves removed from or denied staff privileges at local public and private facilities, not because of who they were, but because these institutions as a result of the AMA policy shift now insisted that all D.O.'s, like their M.D. physicians, be members of the county medical society. Osteopathic practitioners in these states argued that they had no realistic choice but to comply. In the floor debate in the house, a number of other delegations brought out the fact that they too encountered the same allopathic hospital maneuver, but had overcome the problem by seeking and receiving legislative and judicial relief. When Iowa delegates admitted that they had not exhausted their legal options, much of whatever sentiment there was for their measure evaporated. Pennsylvania thereupon withdrew its proposal and the 1968 policy as amended in 1969 was reaffirmed. Another effort at overturning the established rule was made in 1973, but it met a similar fate.[30]

At the end of 1978 only 417 osteopathic practitioners (2.4 percent of all listed D.O.'s) had joined the national AMA.[31] Though it seems that a larger number of D.O.'s are members of local allopathic societies, this figure nonetheless constitutes a small percentage. According to the AOA, dual membership—in it and any political division of the AMA—is rarely encountered. In 1976 it reported that only eleven confirmed cases had been brought to its attention that year.[32] Indeed, total AOA membership continues to be high, and is in fact growing slightly. In 1968, just before the change in AMA policy, 77 percent of all listed D.O.'s belonged to the AOA. In 1978 the figure stood at 80 percent.[33] Clearly the AMA offer of membership produced no outpouring of D.O.'s into its ranks, although it has caused some resentment towards the AOA among those osteopathic practitioners who felt victimized by its position.

The issue of postdoctoral opportunities for D.O.'s in allopathic hospitals presented a far more complex and difficult situation for the AOA. While the association had made considerable strides in upgrading its standards regarding internships and residencies in recent decades, serious weaknesses remained, particularly in some of the specialties. Since D.O. hospitals utilized for such training were typically smaller than those of their M.D. counterparts, the range and depth of experience offered was not always comparable. Also, in some established fields like dermatology and proctology, there were no hospital residencies, only preceptorships, and in other specialties such as psychiatry, few programs existed. Finally, there was the question of those D.O.'s now entering the armed forces and Public Health Service. The only manner in which they could receive formal postdoctoral training while on duty was in federal hospital programs accredited by the AMA.

When the matter first came up before the AOA house in July, 1969, no definitive action was taken. Instead, it was decided to give the AOA Committee on Post-Doctoral Training the authorization to provide applications for nonosteopathic hospital intern and residency programs on an individual basis.[34] This absence of a clear policy led to considerable confusion among the ranks, which was only partly relieved at a joint conference between the AOA board and Associated Colleges representatives held that December. Following this meeting, AOA President J. Scott Heatherington, D.O., addressed a letter to all osteopathic students, faculty, and administrators in which he stated the association's position. "The A.O.A.," he wrote, "recognizes that there are a few highly technical subspecialty fields in which neither the osteopathic nor allopathic approach to health care can be clearly differentiated at this time. Within these limited fields there may be legitimate grounds which enable osteopathic physicians to participate in training under allopathic auspices, but only so long as such sub-specialty training clearly augments, not replaces osteopathic training in the major specialty fields."[35] Students were warned that before they could receive AOA blessing to enter an AMA residency, they had first to complete an AOA-approved rotating internship—that is, one in an osteopathic hospital recognized for that purpose or a federal hospital, "as long as it fits the rules." The next step was to notify the association of the student's intention to enter a nonosteopathic hospital-centered program and have the institution provide a detailed outline of what the course of training would consist of.

At its July, 1970, meeting, the AOA house gave its approval to this basic plan, though again specific criteria under which a candidate might or might not be allowed to take an allopathic residency awaited formulation.[36] For some specialties such as general surgery and internal medicine, where there were a sufficient number of residency programs in osteopathic institutions to meet the needs of D.O. postgraduates, both the AOA and the hospitals feared that these programs might be bypassed unless further restrictions upon allopathic appointments were established. Consequently, in 1970 and 1971, the respective specialty boards in these and other fields began to change their certification requirements to insist that one or more years had to be spent in an osteopathic hospital residency before a student could be given credit for nonfederal allopathic training. Finally, after much delay, AOA policy had taken form.

The optimistic prediction within organized medicine that there would be a mass defection of D.O.'s from AOA-approved postdoctoral programs was not fulfilled, although in the first few years the number of new osteopathic physicians entering nonmilitary AMA programs upon graduation was certainly significant. According to AOA-released data, 12.2 percent of the class of 1970 followed this route.[37] Data subsequently collected (table 3) suggests that this figure remained stable through 1973, when it was 12.3 percent, although thereafter the total began to drop: 9.0 percent in 1974, 3.0 percent in 1975, and 3.3 percent in 1976—this despite the fact that more allopathic hospitals were opening up their programs to D.O.'s. As far as the total number of osteopathic physicians training in AMA-inspected hospital pro-

TABLE 3
Osteopathic Graduates (1972-76) Completing
an AOA-Approved Internship One Year after Graduation

| | | Completing AOA-Approved Internship | | | |
| | | In AOA Hospital | | In Federal Hospital | |
| Year of Graduation | Number of Graduates | Number | % | Number | % |
|---|---|---|---|---|---|
| 1972 | 484 | 373 | 77.1 | 49 | 10.1 |
| 1973 | 650 | 486 | 74.8 | 66 | 10.1 |
| 1974 | 587 | 457 | 77.8 | 74 | 12.6 |
| 1975 | 698 | 603 | 86.4 | 74 | 10.6 |
| 1976 | 809 | 704 | 87.0 | 62 | 7.7 |

| | Entering Non-AOA-Approved Internship | | | | Licensed without Internship | | No Information | |
| | In Allopathic Programs | | In Osteopathic Programs | | | | | |
| Year of Graduation | Number | % | Number | % | Number | % | Number | % |
|---|---|---|---|---|---|---|---|---|
| 1972 | 56 | 11.6 | 2 | 0.4 | 4 | 0.8 | 0 | ... |
| 1973 | 80 | 12.3 | 6 | 0.9 | 6 | 0.9 | 6 | 0.9 |
| 1974 | 53 | 9.0 | 2 | 0.3 | 0 | ... | 1 | 0.2 |
| 1975 | 21 | 3.0 | 0 | ... | 0 | ... | 0 | ... |
| 1976 | 27 | 3.3 | 0 | ... | 0 | ... | 16 | 2.0 |

*Source:* American Association of Colleges of Osteopathic Medicine, *Final Report of the Osteopathic Medical Manpower Information Project* (Washington, D.C., 1977), p. 40.

grams, including those approved by the AOA, a similar pattern may be seen (table 4). The figure rose rapidly each year until 1974, when it began a steady decline which continued through 1977. Meanwhile, the number of residents in osteopathic hospitals made a modest gain between the 1972-73 and 1976-77 contract periods.[38]

Three principal reasons may be offered as to why the large break anticipated by the AMA had not occurred. First, most D.O. students and recent graduates perceived that their postgraduate programs were by and large satisfactory, that the training they would receive was comparable to that available in an allopathic hospital. Second, some prospective trainees believed they would be looked down upon or discriminated against in an M.D. environment. And third, some who wanted to enter an AMA program were fearful of possible AOA disciplinary actions should they not follow its guidelines. One reason why a decline in osteopathic participation in AMA programs occurred after 1973 appears to be a landmark Arizona Court of Appeals decision handed down that same year concerning a D.O. with strictly allopathic postdoctoral credentials who had been denied a medical

TABLE 4
D.O. Physicians in AMA-Approved Programs, 1969-77

| Year, as of September 1 | Interns | Residents | Postgraduates |
|---|---|---|---|
| 1969 | 23 | . . . | 23 |
| 1970 | 117 | 102 | 219 |
| 1971 | 123 | 236 | 359 |
| 1972 | 128 | 427 | 555 |
| 1973 | 128 | 480 | 608 |
| 1974 | 114 | 444 | 558 |
| 1975 | . . . | . . . | . . . |
| 1976 | 61 | 354 | 415 |
| 1977 | 63 | 386 | 449 |

*Source:* "Medical Education in the United States," *Journal of the American Medical Association* 218 (1971): 1247-48; 222 (1972): 1011-12; 226 (1973): 945; 238 (1977): 2790-92; 240 (1978): 2842-44.

*Note:* Programs included military internships and residencies as well as fellowships in nonmilitary hospitals approved by the AOA.

license by the state board of osteopathic examiners on the grounds that he had not served a one-year rotating internship in a hospital program approved by the AOA as required by law. The D.O., backed by the AMA, brought suit claiming that training under the latter's auspices was equivalent and thus should be accepted. The court, however, turned aside this argument and upheld the board's decision. Since at least thirteen other state boards, including the osteopathic strongholds of Michigan, Pennsylvania, Florida, and Oklahoma, were covered by similarly worded statutes, some students who had planned to bypass the AOA-approved routes undoubtedly thought better of the idea.[39]

Though more than a dozen years have elapsed since the AMA inaugurated its osteopathic postgraduate policy, the sociological impact of this change remains difficult to assess. Clearly it has not resulted in the destruction of the AOA program. Still, the number of D.O.'s who have thus far entered internships and residencies in allopathic hospitals (whether AOA approved or unapproved) is not inconsiderable, and this may be serving to undermine the ideology of separateness. On the other hand, the AOA believes that many D.O.'s upon completion of allopathic fellowships in specialty and sub-specialty areas in which the profession has been weak will return to D.O. institutions where they will establish practices and proceed to set up their own teaching programs. This would obviate the need for future outside training, thus making the profession truly self-contained. Many allopathically educated D.O.'s, it would appear, are returning, but more time must pass and additional data must be gathered to analyze this trend adequately.

One of the justifications given by the California delegation to explain the decision to merge with the CMA was that the osteopathic profession was not growing. As a result, the prospects for it becoming socially visible were not good. Indeed, if one surveys the number of graduates produced by the colleges each year prior to 1962, no pattern of continuous expansion can be discerned, only ups and downs related to entrance requirements, economic conditions, and war (see the Appendix). What gains there were in the total number of listed D.O.'s during this period were simply a reflection of the fact that as an occupational group, osteopathic physicians were getting older. Now, with one fewer college, some two thousand fewer practitioners, and a loss of between ninety and one hundred new graduates each year, organized osteopathy saw the necessity not only of replenishing its ranks, but of going well beyond its premerger totals with respect to schools and. practitioners.

In their struggle the D.O.'s were considerably aided by a number of outside factors. Throughout the 1950s claims were being made that there either was, or soon would be, a serious shortage of practicing physicians in the United States since the number of medical schools and graduates was not keeping pace with the postwar growth in population. With the issuance of two Department of Health, Education, and Welfare studies, the so-called Bayne-Jones (1958) and Bane (1959) reports, which lent weight to these conclusions, attention soon shifted to what the federal government could do to eliminate the perceived problem. This, along with concern about the overall quality of medical training, led to the passage of the Health Professions Educational Act of 1963 (Public Law 88-1929), which authorized a program of matching federal funds for construction and improvement of medical schools, together with a program of making loans to students in medicine, osteopathy, and dentistry. Amendments to this act two years later (Public Law 89-290) established a scholarship program, and all of the aforementioned provisions were later included in the Health Manpower Act of 1968 (Public Law 90-490). Federal aid to osteopathic as well as to other professional schools would be further increased with the signing into law of the Comprehensive Health Manpower Training Act of 1971 (Public Law 92-157), which raised support levels for construction, replaced institutional grants with capitation grants to stimulate further enrollment gains, authorized special project monies, and broadened student loan provisions.[40] From fiscal year 1965 through 1976, the Chicago, Des Moines, Kansas City, Kirksville, and Philadelphia schools received a combined total of $65.8 million through these specific programs.[41]

Other new sources of funding were made available. The legislatures of Pennsylvania (1966), Illinois (1970), and Iowa (1973) passed bills inaugurating

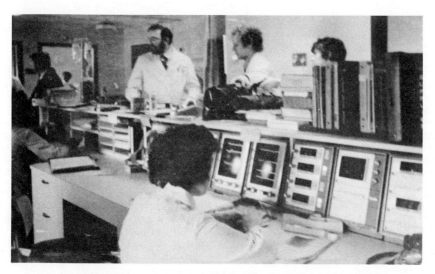

*View from nurses' station at Chicago Osteopathic Hospital (1975).
Courtesy of the Chicago Osteopathic Medical Institutions.*

ongoing educational assistance programs to their respective colleges of osteopathic medicine, in addition to authorizing separate grants for new construction. Further assistance was also secured for the first time from major philanthropic foundations, as well as from the pharmaceutical houses. Increased support from traditional sources also helped. Between 1961-62 and 1974-75, the Osteopathic Progress Fund, supported by D.O.'s in the field, channeled slightly over $16 million into the schools, while the colleges themselves roughly tripled their tuition. In a federally sponsored study published in 1974, it was found that while the median level of sampled D.O. schools was still lower than that of sampled M.D. institutions, all osteopathic colleges examined were now inside the total range of M.D. schools studied with respect to the amount of money each spent per student for educational purposes.[42]

Several significant improvements were made within these five colleges between the time of the merger and the late 1970s. First, the qualifications of their students steadily rose. During the 1958-59 academic year, 72 percent held bachelor's or advanced degrees. In 1968-69, this climbed to 88 percent, and during 1978-79 the total exceeded 95 percent.[43] Second, far more faculty members, particularly full-time staff, were hired. Although differing methods of data collection and organization make accurate comparisons impossible, it is still safe to say that there has been at least a doubling of "full-time" or "whole time" staff since the early 1960s.[44] Finally, equipment and facilities were vastly improved. The Chicago College added two new wings to its existing hospital (1963-70), built a new basic science building (1968), opened

TABLE 5

United States-Trained M.D. and D.O. Physicians and Foreign Medical Graduates
Examination Results before Medical and Composite Licensing Boards,
1955-59 to 1970-72

| Period | U.S. M.D. Examinees | | | U.S. D.O. Examinees | | | Foreign Medical Graduates | | |
|--------|----------|--------|------|----------|--------|------|----------|--------|------|
|        | Examined | Passed | %    | Examined | Passed | %    | Examined | Passed | %    |
| 1955-59 | 30,184  | 28,903 | 95.7 | 1,174    | 954    | 81.2 | 11,192   | 6,787  | 60.6 |
| 1960-64 | 25,992  | 25,360 | 97.6 | 1,980    | 1,678  | 84.7 | 14,534   | 9,959  | 68.5 |
| 1965-69 | 23,364  | 22,321 | 95.5 | 2,135    | 1,887  | 88.4 | 20,800   | 13,242 | 63.7 |
| 1970-72* | 15,922 | 14,368 | 90.2 | 1,401    | 1,241  | 88.6 | 25,725   | 16,477 | 64.1 |

Source: "Medical Licensure Statistics," Journal of the American Medical Association 161 (1956):
341; 164 (1957): 426; 167 (1958): 594; 170 (1959): 573; 173 (1960): 387; 176 (1961): 701; 180 (1962): 847;
184 (1963): 788; 188 (1964): 880; 192 (1965): 858; 196 (1966): 861; 200 (1967): 1058; 204 (1968): 1070; 208
(1969): 2086; 212 (1970): 1875; 216 (1971): 1786; 220 (1972): 1607; 225 (1973): 301.

*Data were not published after 1973. Accuracy of data covering 1973 is in dispute.

a new $12.3 million outpatient clinic (1978), and completed construction of
an $18 million, 200-bed satellite facility (1978). The Kansas City College
added a new library (1968), lecture halls (1971), and a $29 million, 426-bed
teaching hospital (1972). The Philadelphia College built a new campus that
included a 250-bed facility (1968), and the Kirksville school added a new
research building (1963) and completed a major addition to its hospital
(1971), while Des Moines moved its campus to more spacious quarters
(1972).

One indirect measure of improved standards and conditions within these
schools was the overall results of D.O. candidates before M.D. and composite
licensure boards. The most recent data, published by JAMA, would suggest
that there are now no significant statistical differences between U.S. trained
M.D.'s and D.O.'s in passing such examinations (see table 5).

Even more important to the future of the profession, the perceived overall
shortage of physicians helped spur the establishment of new osteopathic
schools, particularly as the existing D.O. colleges had a proven record of
producing a high percentage of the type of doctor most in need, that is,
general practitioners who were most likely to locate in rural and inner city
areas.

The first and most significant battle to establish a new college occurred in
Michigan—now boasting the largest number of osteopathic physicians in
any state. Although hampered by the lack of a school in Michigan, many
D.O.'s were drawn to practice within its borders by an attractice licensure
law, public acceptance, plus the limited licensure of its neighbor Illinois
which discouraged graduates of the Chicago school from staying put. However, with Illinois joining the unlimited licensure ranks in 1955, and later
with the loss of COP&S in 1961, a number of influential Michigan D.O.'s

believed they would have to establish their own institution if they were to increase, much less keep stable, their ranks.

In May, 1963, the Michigan Association of Osteopathic Physicians and Surgeons (MAOP&S) House of Delegates unanimously threw its support behind plans for a new school, which was to be established near East Lansing, home of Michigan State University (MSU). However, when MSU announced shortly thereafter that it was in the process of developing an M.D.-granting institution, the osteopathic college committee, citing a shortage of clinical resources, shifted the location to Pontiac. In March, 1965, a charter was obtained and architects were hired to design the campus.[45]

Meanwhile, representatives and other advocates of the proposed college began lobbying for state aid. They referred legislators to recent surveys conducted by a commission appointed by the governor showing a need for still another medical school since Michigan ranked only twenty-fifth among all states in physician/population ratio.[46] As to why this should be an osteopathic rather than allopathic school, the D.O.'s pointed out that as most of them were general practitioners practicing in underserved areas, they were filling the health care gaps that the M.D.'s were creating. Thus, to solve the physician manpower problem, it made more sense to invest in osteopathic education. These arguments interested the legislature, which in June, 1965, passed a capital outlay bill providing money for a feasibility study. That same month the MAOP&S house assessed each member of the association $2 thousand payable over the next ten years to raise $3 million for the institution, and unveiled plans to amass $5 million elsewhere so as to qualify under the Health Professions Education Act for another $16 million in its two-to-one matching program.[47]

In October, 1966, the Michigan Senate by a vote of twenty-two to seven passed a bill creating the authority for the establishment of a state-supported osteopathic school. Not unexpectedly, the Michigan State Medical Society loudly protested. During hearings on the measure before the House State Affairs Committee the next month, the society's president appeared, forcefully arguing that amalgamation between the two professions was imminent. A state financial school "just for osteopaths," he maintained, would be absurd since at least 75 percent of all D.O.'s in the state favored merger. This assertion was vigorously rebutted by MAOP&S representatives. With no concrete data available for the committee to determine the accuracy of either contention, it decided to commission a confidential mail ballot of all D.O.'s and M.D.'s practicing in Michigan to see how they actually felt. The results, released in early 1967, were unambiguous. To the question "Do you believe amalgamation of allopathy and osteopathy would be in the best interests of the state?" 87.3 percent of the D.O.'s who responded said "no." On the question "Should the state give support to the osteopathic school?" 93.3 percent of the D.O.'s answered "yes." Results from the M.D.'s polled revealed opposite responses in approximately the same proportions. With this new information, the house committee voted ten to one in favor of the College Authority.[48]

Organized medicine, however, did not give up. When the measure came before the full house for consideration in mid-1967 it lobbied intensively and successfully for the bill's defeat, seeing it fail by a margin of only two votes. The legislature, though, had not closed the door on the project, having already allocated another $50 thousand for further study and development. The following year it appropriated $75 thousand more. Finally in 1969 the question of state support came before the legislature once again. This time the osteopathic forces were much better prepared. They responded well to the objections raised by the medical opposition and helped push their bill through both houses and secure the governor's signature.[49]

Under the new statute, the osteopathic college would become an integral part of one of the three existing state universities. Further details were to be decided by the Michigan Board of Education and agreed to by the board of trustees of that institution. After involved negotiations, Michigan State was chosen and accepted. Meanwhile, the board of trustees of the proposed school had previously voted to press ahead with or without state aid. It had already begun its first class in the fall of 1969 and would start a second the following year in Pontiac, before the whole campus would be transferred to East Lansing, where existing buildings were being remodeled for its use. The new Michigan State University College of Osteopathic Medicine (MSU-COM) would share some facilities with the M.D.-granting school now on campus—the College of Human Medicine—but each would be governed by a separate budget and administration. While each would use the same pool of basic science faculty, classes for D.O. and M.D. students would be held separately.[50]

The establishment of MSU-COM was significant in at least three major respects. It was the first new school of osteopathic medicine to be founded in several decades, thus helping to show that the profession was not content with merely maintaining its existing number of colleges and graduates; second, it was the first university-based osteopathic school, thus allowing the entire profession to achieve greater status in the academic community; and third, having a D.O. and M.D. college exist side-by-side on the same campus gave visible expression to the contention by organized osteopathy that the two medical professions were separate but equal.

At the same time that Michigan D.O.'s were making plans for their new school, osteopathic practitioners in Texas were working towards the same end. Enrolling its first class in the fall of 1970, the Texas College of Osteopathic Medicine (TCOM) began inauspiciously, housed initially on the top two floors of Fort Worth Osteopathic Hospital. However, the following year more suitable facilities for basic science instruction were obtained and utilized. Although founded as a private institution, TCOM began receiving some state aid in 1971, and the next year it signed a contract with North Texas State University (NTSU) in Denton for the use of classrooms, faculty, laboratories, and offices. In 1973 state assistance was significantly increased with the passage of an appropriations bill providing TCOM with capitation funds—$11,625 for each bona fide Texas resident enrolled. Two years later a formal agreement was negotiated and signed under which TCOM would become a public institution under the control of the Board of Regents of NTSU. Thus the profession had its second university-affiliated medical school.[51]

Given the successful efforts of Michigan and Texas, D.O. groups in other states began pushing in earnest for their own institutions. The next to be established were the Oklahoma College of Osteopathic Medicine and Surgery of Tulsa and the West Virginia School of Osteopathic Medicine of Greenbriar, both opening in 1974. In the case of Oklahoma, the legislature was impressed by what D.O.'s were already accomplishing in the state in terms of providing medical services in high-priority need areas and was thus willing to expand their role by creating a free-standing public college.[52] In West Virginia, on the other hand, D.O.'s had made comparatively little impact on health care delivery, since there were only some seventy active practitioners. Nevertheless, a determined West Virginia Osteopathic Society, recognizing the dire need for more physicians in the Appalachian region, decided that they were best able to fill the gap. It purchased and remodeled a former military academy and began operations on a limited budget, backed by the necessary, although reluctant, AOA approval and the blessing and support of federal agencies that saw the school as an important experiment in increasing physician manpower in economically depressed areas. The West Virginia legislature soon agreed, and the following year the institution was converted from a private to a free-standing public college.[53]

The drive to create more schools continued. In 1975 the Ohio legislature passed a bill authorizing the establishment of a state osteopathic school at Ohio University, which opened its doors the next year.[54] In 1977 two more colleges began operation: the New Jersey School of Osteopathic Medicine of the College of Medicine and Dentistry, a state institution; and the New York College of Osteopathic Medicine, a private school affiliated with the New York Institute of Technology.[55] In 1978 another two schools were established: the New England College of Osteopathic Medicine of Biddeford, Maine, a component of what is now New England University; and the College of Osteopathic Medicine of the Pacific, a private, nonuniversity affiliated school based in Pomona, California, made possible in part by a 1974 state supreme court ruling which overturned that section of the merger legislation which barred any new osteopathic licensing in California.[56] Buoyed up by their success, California D.O.'s who had remained loyal to the profession vowed to multiply their small numbers quickly and once again make osteopathic medicine a significant part of the health resources of the state.[57]

Thus between 1968 and 1978 the number of osteopathic schools rose from five to fourteen—an incredible leap in so short a period. These new institutions, along with increases in already established osteopathic colleges, brought the level of enrollment far beyond the premerger average. In 1960-61 there were 1,944 students; by 1977-78 this number stood at 3,916. While there were 506 graduates in 1961, there were 964 in 1978 (see the Appendix). The loss of the ex-D.O.'s in California from the ranks of all listed osteopathic practitioners was also more than made up for. The AOA directory premerger figure of 13,923 in 1961 was reached and surpassed in 1973. As of 1978 there were 17,036 listed D.O.'s. According to recent projections based on the then existing number of schools, by 1990 there will be approximately thirty thousand active osteopathic physicians and surgeons.[58]

To most D.O.'s across the country, particularly those who had been in practice at the time of the California merger, all of this has had a significant psychological impact. The college boom, along with the success of organized osteopathy in withstanding AMA pressure for absorption, demonstrated in their minds that their profession was not on the wane. Indeed, in their view, osteopathic medicine appeared to be embarking upon the most fruitful period of its history.

# CHAPTER TEN

# *The Present and the Future*

In many respects, osteopathic medicine does appear to be entering a new phase. One indicator of this is that its longstanding battle to overcome discriminatory practice acts is just about won. With Mississippi in 1973 passing new legislation, and with the California Supreme Court the following year ruling certain provisions of the merger there unconstitutional, D.O.'s finally became eligible for unlimited licensure throughout the fifty states. Two other indicators of this transition are the university affiliation of six of the colleges and their achievement of parity with M.D. schools in terms of the amount of money spent for the training of students.

Where osteopathic medicine is heading, however, is by no means clear. Its recent tremendous growth on the undergraduate level has caused considerable new problems, and some of the issues that have dogged the movement for decades, most notably the role osteopathic structural diagnosis and manipulative therapy should play in total patient care, as well as the dilemmas of status inconsistency and social invisibility, continue to pose considerable threats to its viability as a separate profession. How organized osteopathy deals with this set of circumstances as it heads into the 1980s may be pivotal in determining its future course.

## *Asymmetrical Expansion*

The astonishing increase in the number of osteopathic schools within the past decade has generally been applauded within the profession, but the consequences of this growth have not all been welcomed. One problem has been a sharp tightening of the supply of qualified instructors. While basic science faculty per se has not been especially difficult to secure in the current marketplace, those Ph.D.'s who have already been exposed to and are interested in pursuing teaching and research interests along osteopathic lines are not numerous and have been much in demand. So too have been D.O. staff in most clinical fields. The profession did not systematically plan for the expansion and therefore was unprepared to deal with the shortage of qualified physician instructors. Unlike M.D.-granting schools, which have long encouraged their students to enter careers in research, teaching, and administration, D.O. colleges narrowly focused on turning out practitioners and had no established institutional mechanisms for helping their students follow alternative pathways. Thus as new colleges were established, D.O. institutions were placed in a bind, with the result that a significant number of inexperienced physicians had to be pressed into academic service. Recognizing the problem, some schools have begun to build for the future, searching out and encouraging teaching prospects among their students, as well as establishing special programs to entice basic scientists to enroll for a D.O. degree. Accordingly, this problem seems to be slowly being resolved. However, if the number of schools continues to increase dramatically, the profession is likely to face a long-term problem.[1] (At the time of this writing, a fifteenth school, the Southeastern College of Osteopathic Medicine, located in Florida, is just beginning operations.)

Far more serious is the challenge undergraduate expansion has had and will continue to have for the D.O. internship. In recent decades a greater division has occurred between the allopathic and osteopathic professions over the substance of the first year of postdoctoral education. The number of AMA-approved rotating internships (that is, programs where interns divide their time between several major departments) has been steadily declining over the years in favor of either mixed internships (which are rotating but place emphasis on a specialty) or straight internships (which for all practical purposes are the first year of specialty training). In the 1964-65 school year 50 percent of all AMA-approved internships were rotating; by 1973-74 the percentage had dropped to only 19 percent.[2] The rationale behind this trend is that the mixed and straight internships allow the graduate who wants to specialize to spend more time and thus gain greater experience in his or her own chosen field. All AOA-approved internships, on the other hand, whether they be in osteopathic or federal hospitals, have been and continue to be rotating. Interns must spend three months in both internal medicine and surgery and one month in both obstetrics/gynecology and general practice. There must also be exposure in anesthesiology, pathology, pediatrics, and radiology. The reasoning underlying the rotating internship is that, whether the D.O. becomes a general practitioner or a specialist, he or she must be adequately prepared to take care of the "entire patient" and treat any emergency case or condition that presents itself.[3]

During the 1960s the AOA was able to strengthen its internship program requirements. At the beginning of the decade the minimum number of beds necessary for an osteopathic hospital to become eligible for interns was forty-five. In 1964 it was raised to sixty, and in 1968 to one hundred. Although serving to decrease the number of institutions able to participate, the new standards were not expected to create any major problems as long as first, the number of graduates showed only moderate growth; second, existing D.O. hospitals continued to increase their capacity; and third, new facilities were built.

However, in the 1970s, with the establishment of new schools, the viability of the AOA internship program began to be sorely tested. Between 1972 and 1975 the number of graduates rose from 484 to 698, a 44.2 percent increase. The number of beds in those AOA hospitals participating in the program during the corresponding period rose from 12,626 to 14,061, a 10.6 percent rise. In 1972-73, 62.7 percent of all available internship positions were filled. During 1975-76, the figure stood at 86.3 percent. Projections made at that time based on the number of students then expected to graduate in the coming years who would not be entering federal internships and on the then-current rate of new internship positions revealed that there would be fifty more graduates than available slots in 1977-78, seventy-three in 1978-79, and eighty-three in 1979-80.[4] Unless action was taken to prevent this expected shortfall, there might well be a stampede by graduates into non-AOA-approved allopathic programs.

In 1975 the AOA house adopted guidelines submitted by the Bureau of Professional Education which would allow "consortia arrangements" wherein two or more osteopathic hospitals—either because each hospital did not have enough beds or the required organized departments—could pool their resources to become eligible for interns. Two years later the house adopted an amended format for the rotation of interns on an elective basis through departments of hospitals not accredited by the AOA and for the first time approved the utilization of joint-staff or combined-staff hospitals that were willing to apply for AOA accreditation. These institutions would be required to have an adequate D.O. population in the four major departments and meet other specific criteria.[5] As a result of these changes as well as the establishment of a new formula for basing the number of interns approved for each hospital more on the basis of outpatient services than bed capacity, the AOA has so far been able to create a sufficient number of new internships for all of its nonfederal-bound graduates.[6] However, whether this will continue is problematical. In 1979 there were 1,004 new D.O.'s; by 1989 the number, based on the projections made by the then-existing fourteen schools, will be 1,844—an increase of 84 percent (see table 6).[7]

Complicating the D.O.'s' efforts has been an ever-increasing government monitoring and control of all significant hospital construction. Approximately one-half of the states, believing there was a surplus number of patient beds, which meant duplication of services and, more importantly, rising expenditures for which taxpayers were liable through Medicare and Medicaid, enacted certificate-of-need laws forcing hospitals to submit any major expansion plans to designated public agencies for approval. In all but a few of these laws, passed in the 1960s and early 1970s, there was no provision

TABLE 6
Projected Graduating Class Size for Osteopathic Colleges

| School | 1978-79 | 1979-80 | 1980-81 | 1981-82 | 1982-83 | 1983-84 |
|---|---|---|---|---|---|---|
| Chicago | 94 | 98 | 94 | 96 | 124 | 124 |
| Michigan State | 95 | 90 | 123 | 31 | 115 | 120 |
| Pomona | 0 | 0 | 0 | 36 | 54 | 60 |
| Des Moines | 171 | 174 | 177 | 180 | 186 | 186 |
| Kansas City | 146 | 149 | 157 | 164 | 160 | 184 |
| Kirksville | 120 | 122 | 126 | 130 | 132 | 132 |
| New England | 0 | 0 | 0 | 36 | 56 | 60 |
| New Jersey | 0 | 0 | 23 | 29 | 32 | 32 |
| New York | 0 | 0 | 35 | 54 | 66 | 78 |
| Oklahoma | 68 | 81 | 81 | 81 | 86 | 86 |
| Ohio | 0 | 22 | 33 | 49 | 48 | 60 |
| Philadelphia | 199 | 203 | 207 | 208 | 208 | 208 |
| Texas | 69 | 72 | 74 | 83 | 84 | 88 |
| West Virginia | 42 | 48 | 52 | 59 | 61 | 60 |
| Total | 1,004 | 1,059 | 1,182 | 1,236 | 1,412 | 1,478 |

| School | 1984-85 | 1985-86 | 1986-87 | 1987-88 | 1988-89 | 1989-90 |
|---|---|---|---|---|---|---|
| Chicago | 124 | 124 | 124 | 124 | 124 | 124 |
| Michigan State | 120 | 120 | 120 | 125 | 125 | 125 |
| Pomona | 72 | 72 | 90 | 100 | 100 | 100 |
| Des Moines | 192 | 200 | 200 | 200 | 200 | 200 |
| Kansas City | 208 | 224 | 236 | 250 | 250 | 250 |
| Kirksville | 132 | 132 | 132 | 132 | 132 | 132 |
| New England | 72 | 96 | 112 | 125 | 125 | 125 |
| New Jersey | 48 | 48 | 60 | 60 | 72 | 72 |
| New York | 90 | 102 | 108 | 108 | 108 | 108 |
| Oklahoma | 96 | 96 | 100 | 100 | 100 | 100 |
| Ohio | 60 | 78 | 78 | 100 | 100 | 100 |
| Philadelphia | 208 | 208 | 208 | 208 | 208 | 208 |
| Texas | 88 | 96 | 112 | 125 | 125 | 125 |
| West Virginia | 68 | 68 | 72 | 75 | 75 | 75 |
| Total | 1,578 | 1,664 | 1,752 | 1,832 | 1,844 | 1,844 |

*Source:* Gerald A. Faverman, "The Decade Ahead, A Mighty Challenge," *The D.O.* 19 (April 1979): 76.

for separate osteopathic consideration. Thus some D.O. hospitals operating at near or full capacity were apparently refused permission and money to undertake new construction because M.D. hospitals located in the same community remained underutilized. The AOA charged that this denied the osteopathic patient the type of care he or she desired and served to discriminate unfairly against D.O. institutions, since they were so few in number (approximately three percent of all hospitals).[8] In 1974 Congress passed the National Health Planning and Resources Development Act, which established a network of Health Systems Agencies throughout the country to regulate new construction and equipment expenditures. The AOA lobbied intensively, but unsuccessfully, to have this legislation mandate that Health Systems Agencies make separate evaluations "of the availability of both osteopathic and allopathic facilities and services within a community." Finally, in late 1979, after continuous pressure from the D.O. community, an amendment with language to this effect was signed into law. Whether this measure will be fully implemented will be quite important to the continued cohesion and solidarity of the profession, for if their hospitals are not allowed to expand significantly, and the profession is not allowed to build new ones, many D.O.'s will be forced to seek staff appointments at nonosteopathic institutions—independent of other factors.[9]

## Osteopathy's Lesion

According to some recent studies the current level of O.M.T. use is not particularly high. In 1972 the independent journal *Osteopathic Physician* published the results of a mailed questionnaire returned by 234 D.O.'s (47.3 percent of those sampled) located in ten states across the country. Asked, "On what percent of your patients do you make use of manipulation?" 66.2 percent said under 50 percent, with 37.1 percent responding under 20 percent. However, the actual use may be even lower. In the 1974 national ambulatory medical care survey carried out by the National Center for Health Statistics, it was estimated, based on its sample, that of 53.5 million patient visits during the year to office-based D.O.'s, fewer than 9.1 million (or less than 17 percent) included O.M.T.[10]

The increasing compartmentalization of manipulation to treating localized musculoskeletal complaints such as "back problems," muscle strains, and joint adhesions has caused considerable consternation among those who believe that the modality has a far greater degree of suitability and effectiveness and who realize that its utilization is the principal feature of the D.O.'s' practice that makes it distinctive and gives meaning to the ideology of professional autonomy. Speaking to this issue, Spencer G. Bradford, D.O. of the Philadelphia College, has noted:

> The major contribution of osteopathic medicine to clinical practice arises in part from the recognition of the fact that unimpeded physiologic and bio-chemical functioning of the musculoskeletal system is necessary in the body's effort to maintain homeostasis and optimum health. The modern clinical pre-occupation with etiology, pathogenesis, and biochemical antidisease warfare tends to leave out of consideration the vehicular medium for these infectious and chemical processes: the structure of man himself. Osteopathic theory takes note of the preponderance of somatic tissues and the constant presence of mechanical stress and strain in this human structure, which may play a major

role in its efforts to carry out optimally its function in aiding the body's homeostatic processes. The profession's major contribution to clinical practice, therefore, has been the development of logical and effective means for improving body structure and mechanics under the conditions of pathophysiologic disturbances. Anything that is done to produce more normal structure will enhance the physiologic response of the whole patient. Regardless of the pathogenesis in any given instance the musculoskeletal somatic system is involved and should be evaluated and then treated according to the indications and findings.[11]

This orientation fit in nicely with the ideology of holistic medicine which was then gaining popularity among professionals and lay people.

In recent years efforts have been undertaken to instill in members of the profession a more inclusive view of the role of O.M.T. On the undergraduate level the teaching of courses in osteopathic fundamentals appears to have been considerably improved. Prior to 1960 there were few full-time professors in departments of Osteopathic Principles and Practice (O.P.&P.), and much of the teaching load was in the hands of unpaid volunteer faculty. As previously noted, what monies the schools were able to raise by the Osteopathic Progress Fund and other sources went into supporting those departments and those areas—notably the basic sciences—which had a direct bearing on the ability of their students to pass outside licensing examinations. Consequently, while there appeared to be some outstanding instructors in O.P.&P. during this period, they worked under a considerable financial and educational handicap. After 1960, however, these departments, through endowments and general college funds, were gradually able to build up a corps of full-time professors chosen on the basis of merit rather than on that of the possession of spare time. Nevertheless, this in itself has not been enough, for osteopathic principles and practices, and specifically osteopathic manipulative therapy, have not as yet been satisfactorily integrated throughout the clinical portion of the medical students' experience. Currently most students, after being taught when and under what conditions manipulative intervention is indicated during the first half of the curriculum, are then placed in an environment where it is simply not employed. Obviously this does not enhance the osteopathic medical student's belief in and practice of O.M.T.

After the California merger, the AOA once again began tackling the problem of the diminishing use of O.M.T. in osteopathic hospitals. In 1966 the Board of Trustees passed a resolution requiring a "committee to be established in each accredited institution composed of representatives of each organized department to evaluate the utilization of distinctive osteopathic methods in hospital practice and recommend means of improved application."[12] While these committees have been formed and must meet once each month, they have, it would seem, achieved little, if anything, in the way of promoting the recording of structural findings on patients' charts and seeing to it that O.M.T. where applicable is given. At present the great majority of osteopathic institutions upon inspection by the AOA for the purpose of accreditation are consistently cited for their failure in this regard, but as this deficiency alone has never been used as the sole basis, or for that matter even a significant criterion, for determining whether or not accreditation should be granted, most hospitals have simply disregarded AOA admonishments.

This situation, though, may be changing as an unanticipated consequence of the surplus beds problem. In 1973 local health care planners advised the three hospitals of Waterville, Maine, that they believed only one institution was necessary to accommodate the needs of the community. The sole osteopathic institution, faced with the prospect of being forced to shut down or merge with the other two, decided to prove it should remain open by demonstrating it was distinctive. Recognizing that O.M.T. was no longer a regular feature of patient care, its Board of Trustees hired a "Director of Osteopathic Medicine," a D.O. who would provide structural diagnosis and manipulative therapy on a strictly referral basis. The results of the program surprised even its originators. Patients who were given O.M.T. (from 20 to 30 percent of all admissions) seemed highly satisfied with this service and, most importantly, came to expect and indeed ask for such therapy in other than local musculoskeletal disorders. Furthermore, a rough retrospective study suggested that the patients who were treated manipulatively in a number of disease categories were able to be discharged earlier than those who were not, thus raising the interest of third-party carriers concerned with reducing costs. Finally, the overall occupancy rate of the hospital rose. This was attributed in part to new patients who were attracted by the favorable word-of-mouth publicity the new service received.[13] Given the apparent success of this experiment on many different levels, some forty other osteopathic hospitals within the past few years have copied or are in the process of introducing the Waterville model.

With the increasing competition between hospitals for patients, with government insisting upon cutting expenses, and with D.O. facilities needing to prove their distinctiveness, it is quite possible that far more osteopathic facilities and even joint-staff institutions will follow suit. What effect this program might have on the overall use of O.M.T. is difficult to say. While its advocates hope that the various hospital staff members, as well as graduates and undergraduate trainees, seeing the results that O.M.T. can achieve, will begin to employ it themselves, it is also possible that O.M.T., at least in the hospital environment, will simply become regarded as but another specialized task, to be performed only by the highly proficient.[14]

Even assuming the success of this program in osteopathic hospitals, there is still the question of what the profession can do to encourage distinctive osteopathic care in federal facilities in which D.O.'s serve. One can speculate that if the number of osteopathic practitioners in such institutions continues to increase, as it has in recent years, the AOA might eventually be able to go beyond its present role of simply approving federal internships and residencies to actually accrediting the facilities themselves, notwithstanding the present Joint Commission on Accreditation of Hospitals inspection. This would at least place these institutions under the same guidelines covering osteopathic hospitals vis-à-vis the recording of structural findings and the use of manipulative therapy by the D.O. staff. Yet even if this accrediting process is started, its relevance towards distinctive osteopathic care would depend on whether the AOA is prepared to enforce its own rules.

While the utilization of distinctly osteopathic procedures rests in part upon such factors as how much training the D.O. student and postgraduate receives in them, patient acceptance and demand for their use, and the need to conform to association policy, the most crucial seems to be the practitioner's belief in their efficacy in a given situation. Modern osteopathic graduates are far less likely than were their predecessors to accept the validity of O.M.T. on the basis of faith, or philosophy. They enter school with a far stronger background in scientific method and a more critical eye towards evidence. To date, however, scientific research under osteopathic auspices has at best only provided a logical rationale for the use of O.M.T. in other than local nonmusculoskeletal conditions. The studies on segmental facilitation, and the relatively new research beginning in the 1960s on the trophic function of nerves to which Korr and other osteopathic investigators have made a significant contribution, can explain some of the neurophysiologic mechanisms that may account for "the lesion" and its possible role in the disease process, but it remains to be shown experimentally precisely what the relationship is.[15] Even more necessary, it would appear, is a commitment by the profession to go beyond the anecdotal and conduct controlled clinical studies on the effects of manipulative therapy in treating patients. As previously noted, manipulation presents inherently greater problems with respect to establishing controls than does a pharmacologic agent. However, this does not mean that valid clinical trials utilizing O.M.T. cannot be designed and carried out. Indeed, it is simply not enough, either for skeptical potential clients or for that matter its younger practitioners, for the profession to say "O.M.T. works." Given the fact that several of the new schools are university based, the profession is now in a suitable position to train D.O.'s as researchers, and a creditable body of clinical literature may thus be created.[16]

Studies carried out over the past decade clearly suggest that a significant proportion of the American people continue to be largely ignorant of the existence of the profession and what its practitioners do—or that they do know and are not duly impressed. In 1969 the *Osteopathic Physician* published the results of a survey sponsored by the Ohio state osteopathic society. Interviews were conducted with residents of Columbus and Dayton, where D.O.'s represented 13 percent and 27 percent of all physicians and surgeons in those cities respectively. In answer to the question, "What is meant by the term Doctor of Osteopathy or Osteopath?" 28 percent of the respondents admitted that they had never heard of either and 10.5 percent confused it with optometrist, optician, chiropractor, or some other non-M.D. practitioner. In the area of education, 35.9 percent of the sample felt D.O.'s had less training than M.D.'s, while 12.6 percent felt the D.O. had more. Choosing which type of practitioner was the most competent, 44.1 percent said the M.D., while only 3.6 percent answered the D.O.[17]

Similarly, in 1974 there appeared a study of occupational prestige differences within the medical specialties and allied health professions which received national public attention when the results were picked up by a Sunday newspaper supplement. M.D. physicians and patients in three Chicago area allopathic hospitals and graduate business students at the University of Chicago were interviewed. Each group was asked how much they personally looked up to all the specialists and allied professionals listed. Of forty-one occupational titles, both the M.D.'s and the allopathic hospital patients ranked the category "osteopath" thirty-seventh, while the business school students placed it slightly higher, at thirty-first.[18] For those who did not know what a given specialist or allied health professional did, a card was handed out describing his or her responsibilities. An "osteopath" was defined as "a physician educated in a school of osteopathy with emphasis on manipulation of bodily organs in addition to therapeutic and surgical treatment." While it is likely that this definition had no appreciable effect on the overall results obtained, the principal researcher's inability adequately to define *osteopathy* is certainly reflective of the general problem which the profession continues to face.[19]

In March, 1981, the AOA released a paper that contained the results of a survey of public attitudes towards medical care and medical professionals which the association itself had underwritten. Of the sample of 1,003 people eighteen years of age and older chosen at random by telephone, slightly under 20 percent reported that they had heard of the abbreviation D.O. in medicine, but when they were asked what it stood for only 50 percent (or approximately 10 percent overall) correctly connected it with a Doctor of

Osteopathy or Osteopathic Medicine. When the entire sample was later asked the open-ended question, "If someone asked you to explain what an osteopathic physician is, what would you say?" the general lack of knowledge became painfully clear. Leading the responses with 17 percent was "bone specialists/bone surgeons/treat bone diseases/tumors/fractures," closely followed by "manipulative therapy/massage bones or muscles like a chiropractor," with 16 percent. Thirteen percent listed "incorrect specialties" and 7 percent said "a chiropractor who can write a prescription or an M.D. who performs manipulative therapy."[20]

The failure to achieve high levels of recognition and respect among the general public is unquestionably the single most important source of discontent within the profession today, and potentially the most explosive. At the present time the number of D.O.'s who are actively in favor of a merger with the AMA appears to be comparatively small; however, there are a greater number who, while wishing to keep the profession autonomous, are in favor of their schools changing the degree awarded to an M.D. and wish to be allowed to list themselves in that manner. They argue that by making these changes there will be no further doubt in the minds of the general public or their patients that they are not "osteopaths" but "physicians and surgeons" who are due all the respect and prestige accorded holders of the M.D. occupational title.[21]

There seems little likelihood that the AOA is about to alter its policy of recognizing the D.O. degree as the sole professional degree to be issued by the accredited colleges. Understanding this, dissident D.O.'s have sought instead to secure the orthodox medical designation independently, through judicial and legislative means. In 1973 a three-judge federal panel approved the right of a Georgia D.O. to describe himself in his practice as an M.D. and be issued an M.D. license by the state composite board of medical examiners. The court's decision was based on the fact that the board was already licensing all foreign medical graduates as M.D.'s although some held D.M., M.B., or other "equivalent" degrees from institutions abroad. As the board could not, in the court's opinion, show "any reasonable basis for its differing treatment of foreign trained physicians and D.O.'s," since both received unlimited licenses to practice medicine, it declared that the board's denial of an M.D. license to a D.O. was "arbitrary and in violation of the Equal Protection Clause of the 14th Amendment."[22] However, nationally no pattern of such decisions can thus far be discerned, as similar actions brought against the composite boards of New York and New Jersey were dismissed in 1978.[23]

Organized medicine appears split over the issue, as reflected in a narrow defeat in 1974 of a resolution introduced into the AMA House of Delegates urging that state medical societies sponsor legislation to allow D.O.'s to use the initials "M.D." in identifying themselves.[24] In practice, most state medical societies have thus far joined with their state osteopathic association counterparts to fight these bills and suits. However, at least one, the California Medical Association, is actively pressing for such a statute. In 1978 their measure was tabled in committee when the governor announced that he would veto it if it passed. An attempt the following year by the state's medical board to accomplish the same purpose was also unsuccessful.[25]

These challenges, particularly those initiated by D.O.'s themselves, pose a vexing dilemma to organized osteopathy. As long as the profession is not able to improve its public image significantly, such efforts will continue to draw supporters. It is not, after all, the M.D. degree in and of itself that seems important to these practitioners, but what the degree represents. Thus if the D.O.'s can gain widespread recognition as competent and distinctive physicians and surgeons through their present designation, some of those who now consider their degree an albatross might change their minds and perhaps even come to see it as giving them a competitive edge over the M.D.'s in the marketplace. Indeed, such a development is expected by many leaders of organized osteopathy. They believe the profession is now growing so rapidly and making such a significant contribution to American health care that it can no longer be ignored by the national media as has been the case up to the present.[26] Furthermore, given its emphasis upon producing the type of practitioners that are perceived to be needed at this time in the United States, its current high standards, and the fact that D.O.'s have "something extra" in their therapeutic armamentarium, the media coverage they will receive should be generally favorable, thus allowing them to receive what they believe is the proper recognition and respect from the public. This, though, remains problematical, and it should be kept in mind that rising expectations as to an improved condition accompanied by the subjectively held belief that change is not happening fast enough may in fact only result in a greater desire for an M.D. degree, or even spur a renewed sentiment in favor of merger.

The present lack of public recognition, along with the other problems of asymmetrical growth and the decline in the use of distinctively osteopathic procedures, all constitute a serious threat to the future of the profession. Nevertheless, one must also consider the past record of the D.O.'s in meeting such challenges. In this regard, AOA editor George Northup, D.O., has aptly observed, "Those who make gloomy predictions erroneously believe that we do not recognize the problems and if we do, are unable to solve them. Our present status, growth and strength are visible proof that we did not concentrate on the negative aspects of our problems but accepted them as creative stimuli to progress. The only really new and added danger is ironically our success. Our greatest danger is that our success will give birth to complacency—and only complacency can do us in. The future of osteopathic medicine is not in the hands of those who oppose us, but rather in the hands of those who believe in it the most."[27]

# *Appendix*

Graduates of AOA-Accredited or -Approved Osteopathic Colleges, 1898-1981

| Academic Year Ending | Schools* | Graduates† |
|---|---|---|
| 1898 | 10 | 171 |
| 1899 | 12 | 332 |
| 1900 | 13 | 514 |
| 1901 | 13 | 649 |
| 1902 | 11 | 629 |
| 1903 | 10 | 562 |
| 1904 | 10 | 533 |
| 1905 | 11 | 535 |
| 1906 | 9 | 410 |
| 1907 | 9 | 271 |
| 1908 | 8 | 178 |
| 1909 | 8 | 277 |
| 1910 | 8 | 318 |
| 1911 | 9 | 353 |
| 1912 | 8 | 393 |
| 1913 | 8 | 342 |
| 1914 | 8 | 378 |
| 1915 | 7 | 382 |
| 1916 | 8 | 392 |
| 1917 | 7 | 463 |
| 1918 | 7 | 305 |
| 1919 | 7 | 159 |
| 1920 | 7 | 164 |
| 1921 | 7 | 205 |
| 1922 | 8 | 160 |
| 1923 | 8 | 334 |
| 1924 | 8 | 376 |
| 1925 | 7 | 410 |
| 1926 | 7 | 444 |
| 1927 | 6‡ | 417 |
| 1928 | 6 | 338 |
| 1929 | 6 | 354 |
| 1930 | 7‡ | 349 |
| 1931 | 6 | 388 |
| 1932 | 6 | 351 |
| 1933 | 6 | 364 |
| 1934 | 6 | 355 |
| 1935 | 6 | 444 |

| Academic Year Ending | Schools* | Graduates† |
|---|---|---|
| 1936 | 6 | 414 |
| 1937 | 6 | 395 |
| 1938 | 6 | 437 |
| 1939 | 6 | 438 |
| 1940 | 6 | 427 |
| 1941 | 6 | 486 |
| 1942 | 6 | 443 |
| 1943 | 7§ | 431 |
| 1944 | 7§ | 346 |
| 1945 | 6 | 261 |
| 1946 | 6 | 213 |
| 1947 | 6 | 176 |
| 1948 | 6 | 144 |
| 1949 | 6 | 202 |
| 1950 | 6 | 373 |
| 1951 | 6 | 427 |
| 1952 | 6 | 427 |
| 1953 | 6 | 462 |
| 1954 | 6 | 449 |
| 1955 | 6 | 459 |
| 1956 | 6 | 467 |
| 1957 | 6 | 442 |
| 1958 | 6 | 438 |
| 1959 | 6 | 467 |
| 1960 | 6 | 427 |
| 1961 | 6 | 506 |
| 1962 | 5 | 362 |
| 1963 | 5 | 362 |
| 1964 | 5 | 354 |
| 1965 | 5 | 395 |
| 1966 | 5 | 369 |
| 1967 | 5 | 405 |
| 1968 | 5 | 427 |
| 1969 | 5 | 427 |
| 1970 | 6 | 432 |
| 1971 | 7 | 472 |
| 1972 | 7 | 485 |
| 1973 | 7 | 650 |
| 1974 | 7 | 587 |
| 1975 | 9 | 698 |
| 1976 | 9 | 809 |
| 1977 | 10 | 891 |
| 1978 | 12 | 964 |
| 1979 | 14 | 1,004 |
| 1980 | 14 | 1,033 |
| 1981 | 14 | 1,194 |

*Sources:* All figures prior to 1958 derived from Josephine L. Seyl, "Doctors by Osteopathic Colleges by Year of Graduation as of November 1, 1957," typescript, American Osteopathic Association Archives, Chicago, n.d. Subsequent figures generated from the records of the AOA Membership Department.

*Note:* From 1898 through 1901 the AOA accepted the list of approved member institutions of the Associated Colleges of Osteopathy.

*Early schools were not given accredited status by the AOA until after they had graduated their first class. Beginning in 1969 the category "provisionally accredited" was used by the AOA to identify those schools that have met the minimum standards for colleges of osteopathic medicine as established by the AOA Board of Trustees and that have entered students but that have not yet graduated a class. For the purpose of this table the number of schools for each year reflects the existence of accredited schools as well as those that would become fully accredited when eligible.

†Total graduates by year as confirmed through records of the Membership and Education departments of the AOA.

‡AOA accreditation of the Massachusetts College of Osteopathy (MCO) was withheld in 1926-27, restored for 1929-30, and withheld again beginning the next year.

§During the 1942-43 and 1943-44 school years, all classes of the MCO were approved by the AOA, and its graduates were eligible for membership in the association, although the school did not receive full accreditation standing. For the purpose of this table, the college and its graduates during these two years have been included in the overall figures. The MCO closed in 1944.

# *Notes*

## Chapter 1: Andrew Taylor Still

1. Andrew T. Still, *The Autobiography of Andrew Taylor Still* (Kirksville: By the author, 1908), p. 18.

2. For an extended description and analysis of the circuit system see William W. Sweet, *Methodism in American History* (Nashville: Abingdon Press, 1954), pp. 143-85. Also of interest is Edward Eggleston, *The Circuit Rider* (New Haven: College and University Press, 1966).

3. Horace Bushnell quoted in Winthrop S. Hudson, *American Protestantism* (Chicago: University of Chicago Press, 1961), p. 92.

4. Still, *Autobiography*, pp. 18, 19-21.

5. Sweet, *Methodism*, p. 158.

6. Roy F. Nichols, "The Kansas-Nebraska Act: A Century of Historiography," *Mississippi Valley Historical Review* 48 (1956): 187-212.

7. Still, *Autobiography*, pp. 58-72. Also see William F. Zornow, *Kansas: A History of the Jayhawk State* (Norman: University of Oklahoma Press, 1957), pp. 67-80.

8. D. W. Wilder, *The Annals of Kansas* (Topeka: Kansas Publishing House, 1886), pp. 409-11; Still, *Autobiography*, pp. 73-81.

9. Still, *Autobiography*, p. 76.

10. See William Norwood, *Medical Education in the United States before the Civil War* (Philadelphia: University of Pennsylvania Press, 1944). According to Bonner, the number of self-taught practitioners in Kansas was quite high: "In the heroic early years of Kansas medicine when settlers were scattered and doctors few, a doctor might almost be defined as anyone who was practicing medicine. No questions were asked if the practitioner brought relief from suffering. Frequently rough in dress and speech, half-literate, without formal training in medicine, the amateur physician was nevertheless on occasion a man of talents" (Thomas Bonner, *The Kansas Doctor* [Lawrence: University of Kansas Press, 1959], p. 11).

11. William G. Rothstein, *American Physicians in the Nineteenth Century: From Sects to Science* (Baltimore: The Johns Hopkins University Press, 1972), pp. 85-87.

12. The makeup of his early medical library has not been completely settled. A letter dated October 29, 1943, from Dr. M. D. Warner, then Dean of the Kirksville College, to American Osteopathic Association editor Ray Hulburt indicates that the school possessed a number of Still's early books, including an unidentified 1845 dispensatory; Johannes Muller's *Elements of Physiology* (Philadelphia: Lea and Blanchard, 1843); Robert Druitt's *Principles and Practice of Modern Surgery* (Philadelphia: Lea and Blanchard, 1842); William Ferguson's *A System of Practical Surgery* (London: J. Churchill, 1842); and Robert Harrison's *The Dublin Dissector* (New York: S. S. and W. Wood, 1858). In the

intervening years many of these books have, unfortunately, disappeared from the school's archives. However, two others have been discovered: Robley Dunglison's *The Practice of Medicine: A Treatise on Special Pathology and Therapeutics,* vol. 2 (Philadelphia: Lea and Blanchard, 1844), and Samuel Cooper's *The First Lines of the Practice of Surgery,* vol. 1 (New York: James and John Harper Printers, 1822).

13. Still, *Autobiography,* pp. 57, 84-85.

14. James Moore Still (1826-1907) received his M.D. from Rush Medical School in 1864. See James Moore Brown and Robert Bell Woodworth, *The Captives of Abb's Valley* (Staunton, Va.: McClure, 1942), p. 48. In an article written for the *Ladies' Home Journal* in 1908 and reprinted in George Webster, ed., *Concerning Osteopathy* (Carthage, New York: Cruikshank and Ellsworth, 1910), pp. 55-65, A. T. Still claimed that he had attended classes at the Kansas City College of Physicians and Surgeons in 1861, just prior to the Civil War. A skeptical reader of the journal the *Osteopathic Physician* requested proof. Its editor, Henry S. Bunting, wrote to Still's son-in-law, George Laughlin, for clarification, who in turn asked Still. The latter thereupon "corrected" himself, saying it was just after the war, in the winter of 1865 and 1866, that he enrolled in the Kansas City school. He furthermore stated that it was for one term only, as he was so thoroughly disgusted with the "outfit" he decided not to return for his diploma. See "Asks If A. T. Still Ever Was a Real Doctor," *Osteopathic Physician* (hereafter *O.P.*) 15 (January 1909): 8. Because of an absence of records, I cannot establish whether Still ever attended. It is a fact, however, that the first medical school established in Kansas City did not open its doors until 1869. See Carrie Whitney, *Kansas City, Missouri: Its History and Its People, 1808-1908,* 2 vols. (Chicago: S. J. Clarke Publishing, 1908) 1:475.

15. In a document dated December 17, 1877, pertaining to his application for an army pension, Still declared, "I was surgeon *but* the adjutant placed me on the role as a hospital steward and was paid as such. The whole reg[iment] will testify to the truthfulness of the statement. I did the duty of surgeon" (Pension File of Andrew T. Still, Chicago, American Osteopathic Association Archives). See also Still, *Autobiography,* p. 186; Andrew T. Still, "Dr. Still's Department," *Journal of Osteopathy* (hereafter *J. Ost.*) 7 (August 1900): 98-99.

16. Saul Jarcho, "John Mitchell, Benjamin Rush, and Yellow Fever," *Bulletin of the History of Medicine* (hereafter *Bull. Hist. Med.*) 31 (1957): 132-36.

17. Lester S. King, "The Bloodletting Controversy: A Study in the Scientific Method," *Bull. Hist. Med.* 35 (1961): 1-13; Rothstein, *American Physicians,* pp. 45-49. As late as 1912 William Osler was still advocating the use of bloodletting in treating pneumonia. See his *The Principles and Practice of Medicine,* 8th ed. (New York: D. Appleton, 1912), pp. 99-100. According to Bonner, bloodletting was used quite extensively in Kansas throughout the 1850s, less so in the 1860s, and rarely in the 1870s. Bonner, *Kansas Doctor,* pp. 20-21.

18. See G. B. Risse, "Calomel and the American Medical Sects during the Nineteenth Century," *Mayo Clinic Proceedings* 48 (1973): 57-64. Also Rothstein, *American Physicians,* pp. 50-60; Bonner, *Kansas Doctor,* p. 21.

19. Risse, "Calomel and American Medical Sects," p. 58.

20. Erwin H. Ackerknecht, "Aspects of the History of Therapeutics," *Bull. Hist. Med.* 36 (1962): 400-412.

21. Jacob Bigelow, *A Discourse on Self-Limited Disease* (Boston: Ticknor and Fields, 1854), p. 4.

22. Oliver Wendell Holmes, *Medical Essays, 1842-1882* (Boston: Houghton Mifflin, 1892), p. 203.

23. Gert H. Brieger, "Therapeutic Conflicts and the American Medical Profession in the 1860s," *Bull. Hist. Med.* 41 (1967): 215-22.

24. Bonner, *Kansas Doctor,* pp. 10-47; 23-30.

25. Andrew T. Still, "Dr. Still's Department," *J. Ost.* 6 (August 1899): 92-93. See also Bonner, *Kansas Doctor,* p. 21.

26. Still, *Autobiography*, pp. 87-88.

27. Ibid., p. 88.

28. See Samuel Thomson, *The New Guide to Health* (Boston: By the author, 1832); Alex Berman, "The Thomsonian Movement and Its Relation to American Pharmacy and Medicine," *Bull. Hist. Med.* 35 (1951): 405-28, 519-33; Rothstein, *American Physicians,* pp. 125-51; Joseph Kett, *The Formation of the American Medical Profession: The Role of Institutions, 1780-1860* (New Haven: Yale University Press, 1968), pp. 97-131.

29. Kett, *Formation of the American Medical Profession,* p. 23.

30. See Martin Kaufman, *Homeopathy in America: The Rise and Fall of a Medical Heresy* (Baltimore: The Johns Hopkins University Press, 1972); Rothstein, *American Physicians,* pp. 152-73, 230-43, 294-301; Kett, *Formation of the American Medical Profession,* pp. 132-64.

31. Holmes, *Medical Essays,* pp. ix-x.

32. Rothstein, *American Physicians,* pp. 237-39.

33. Alexander Wilder, *History of Medicine* (New Sharon, Maine: By the author, 1901), pp. 512-761; J. M. Scudder, "A Brief History of Eclectic Medicine," *Eclectic Medical Journal* 39 (1879): 297-308; Ronald Numbers, "The Making of an Eclectic Physician," *Bull. Hist. Med.* 47 (1973): 155-66; Rothstein, *American Physicians,* pp. 217-29.

34. See the table of students and graduates by sect, from 1850 to 1920, in Rothstein, *American Physicians,* p. 287.

35. Still, "Dr. Still's Department," *J. Ost.* 6 (August 1899): 92-93.

36. For the rise of temperance in Methodism, see Sweet, *Methodism,* pp. 171-72, 241-42, 235. For temperance as a social phenomenon, see Joseph Gusfield, *Symbolic Crusade: Status Politics and the American Temperance Movement* (Urbana: University of Illinois Press, 1963), pp. 13-57.

37. Still, *Autobiography,* p. 83.

38. Richard H. Shryock, "Sylvester Graham and the Popular Health Movement, 1830-1870," *Mississippi Valley Historical Review* 18 (1931): 172-83; 178.

39. Sylvester Graham, *Lectures on the Science of Human Life,* 2 vols. (Boston: Marsh, Capen, Lyon and Webb, 1839).

40. See in particular Marshall Scott Legan, "Hydropathy in America: A Nineteenth-Century Panacea," *Bull. Hist. Med.* 45 (1971): 267-80; also Henry E. Sigerist, "American Spas in Historical Perspective," *Bull. Hist. Med.* 11 (1942): 133-47. Quote is from Legan, p. 274.

41. This story is related on pp. 195-201 of an unpublished, untitled manuscript by his sister Marovia Still Clark which is preserved in the archives of the Kirksville College of Osteopathic Medicine, Kirksville, Missouri.

42. For a brief discussion of those healers who employed stroking earlier, see Vincent Buranelli, *The Wizard from Vienna: Franz Anton Mesmer* (New York: Coward, McCann, and Geoghagen, 1975), pp. 17-25. One contemporary of Mesmer deserving of special mention was the American Elisha Perkins (1741-1799), who employed two metallic rods that he called *tractors* to perform similar cures. Believing that his discovery would benefit acute, infectious disease as well as nervous disorders, Perkins lost his life testing his theory during a yellow fever epidemic in New York. See Jacques M. Quen, "Elisha Perkins, Physician, Nostrum-Vendor or Charlatan?" *Bull. Hist. Med.* 37 (1963): 159-66.

43. Buranelli, *Wizard from Vienna,* pp. 59-132.

44. *Report of Dr. Benjamin Franklin and Other Commissioners Charged . . . with the Examination of the Animal Magnetism* (London: printed for L. Johnson, 1785); Buranelli, *Wizard from Vienna,* pp. 157-68.

45. *Report of the Magnetical Experiments Made by the Commission of the Royal Academy of Paris, Read on the Meetings of June 21st and 28th, 1831, by Mr. Husson, the Reporter,* trans. and intro. Charles Poyen (Boston: D. K. Hitchcock, 1836). James Braid,

*Neurypnology; Or the Rationale of Nervous Sleep: Considered in Relation with Animal Magnetism* (London: J. Churchill, 1843), and idem, *Observations on Trance; Or Human Hibernation* (London: J. Churchill, 1850).

46. Eric T. Carlson, "Charles Poyen Brings Mesmerism to America," *Journal of the History of Medicine* (hereafter *J. Hist. Med.*) 15 (1960): 121-32.

47. Charles Poyen, *Progress of Animal Magnetism in New England* (Boston: Weeks, Jordan, 1837); C. F. Durant, *Exposition; Or a New Theory of Animal Magnetism* (New York: Wiley and Putnam, 1837); W. L. Stone, *Letter to Dr. A. Brigham on Animal Magnetism* (New York: George Dearborn, 1837); A Gentleman from Philadelphia, *The Philosophy of Animal Magnetism* (Philadelphia: Merrihew and Gunn, 1837).

48. For a description of Quimby's practice and differing accounts of his relative impact upon Eddy, see Frank Podmore, *From Mesmer to Christian Science: A Short History of Mental Healing* (New York: University Book, 1963), pp. 250-99; and Robert Peel, *Mary Baker Eddy: The Years of Discovery, 1821-1875* (New York: Holt, Rinehart and Winston, 1966), pp. 146-338. See also Annetta G. Dresser, *The Philosophy of P. P. Quimby* (Boston: George H. Ellis, 1895); Mary Baker Eddy, *Science and Health with Key to the Scriptures* (Boston: First Church of Christ Scientist, 1971).

49. Robert W. Delp, "Andrew Jackson Davis: Prophet of American Spiritualism," *Journal of American History* 20 (1967): 43-57.

50. Andrew Jackson Davis, *The Great Harmonia,* 4 vols. (Boston: Benjamin B. Mussey, 1853) 1: 325-30.

51. See John F. Teahan, "Warren Felt Evans and Mental Healing," *Church History* 48 (1979): 63-80.

52. Warren Felt Evans, *Mental Medicine* (Boston: H. H. Carter, 1885), p. 109. Edwin Dwight Babbitt, *Vital Magnetism* (New York: By the author, 1874). See also James Mack, *Healing by Laying On of Hands* (Boston: Colby and Rich, 1879), pp. 164-71, which contains Babbitt's "Rules for Magnetizers." *Banner of Light* 36 (January 9, 1875): 8. This letter was an appeal for assistance on behalf of the people of Kirksville, who were suffering the effects of a grasshopper invasion. Written by one Henry Durgin and co-signed by Still and three others, it noted, "There are a few workers here [spiritualists?] but we are looked upon as 'crazy' and 'worse than infidels' and any calamity that may fall upon us is construed to be the just judgment of God, for our daring to think and act for ourselves." Whether Still himself was a spiritualist is unclear, however. Nowhere in his published writings did he profess an allegiance to the belief system. In 1903 he did attend a spiritualist meeting in Clinton, Iowa, whereupon he reported back to his students that the spiritualists' views on drugging were similar to his own, but did not otherwise indicate how far his sympathies with them went. *Bulletin of the Axis and Atlas Clubs* 4 (September 1903): 3-7.

53. See in particular Andrew T. Still, *Philosophy of Osteopathy* (Kirksville: By the author, 1899), pp. 44, 48, 57, 65.

54. Still, *Autobiography,* p. 182. Perhaps this idea stemmed from his training as an orthodox physician, for as Bonner has noted of pre-War Kansas practitioners generally, "From the books they had read and the medical colleges they had attended they viewed disease as largely the work of the blood" (Bonner, *Kansas Doctor,* pp. 21-22).

55. Still, *Autobiography,* p. 108.

56. See E. M. Violette, *History of Adair County* (Kirksville: Journal Printing, 1911), p. 343. *North Missouri Register,* March 11, 1875. This notice ran in the *Register* until August of that year. From this time forward Still does not appear to have used the newspapers for advertising purposes.

57. Still registered as a physician and surgeon in Macon County on August 29, 1874. In 1883 he was issued a similar license for the county of Adair. See documents reprinted in Arthur G. Hildreth, *The Lengthening Shadow of Andrew Taylor Still* (Kirksville: Journal Printing, 1942), pp. 294-95.

58. Still, *Autobiography*, p. 112. Pension File of Andrew Taylor Still.

59. E. R. Booth, *History of Osteopathy and Twentieth-Century Medical Practice* (Cincinnati: The Caxton Press, 1924), pp. 505-6.

60. Dr. Percival Potts said of his famous eighteenth-century bonesetting contemporary "Crazy Sally" Mapp, "Even the absurdities and impracticality of her own promises and engagements, were by no means equal to the expectations the credulity of those who ran after her, that is, of all ranks and degrees of people from the lowest laborer up to those of the most exalted rank and station, several of whom not only did not hesitate implicitly the most extravagant assertions of this ignorant, drunken, female savage, but even solicited her company or at least seemed to enjoy her society" (Quoted in C. J. S. Thompson, *The Quacks of Old London* [London: Brentano, 1928], p. 303).

61. James Paget, "Cases That Bonesetters Cure," *British Medical Journal* 1 (January 5, 1867): 1-4.

62. Wharton Hood, *On Bonesetting, So-Called, and Its Relation to the Treatment of Joints Crippled by Injury* (London: Macmillan, 1871), pp. 4, 26-27.

63. Ibid., pp. 149, viii.

64. Robert J. T. Joy, "The Natural Bonesetters with Special Reference to the Sweet Family of Rhode Island," *Bull. Hist. Med.* 28 (1965): 416-41.

65. Douglas Graham, *A Practical Treatise on Massage: Its History, Mode of Application, and Effects* (New York: William Wood, 1884), p. 20.

66. Some bonesetters were apparently active in and around Missouri during this era. One M.D. wrote of an individual claiming to be one of the Rhode Island Sweets working his trade in his near neighborhood. See A. J. Steele, "The Osteopathic Fad," *Transactions of the Medical Association of the State of Missouri* (1895): 343-58.

67. Still, *Autobiography*, pp. 100-101.

68. Homer E. Bailey quoted in Booth, *History of Osteopathy*, p. 32. See also Hildreth, *Lengthening Shadow*, p. 382.

69. Examples of Still's approach to public speaking can be found in his *Autobiography*. See pp. 153-66, 177-81.

70. Harry M. Still quoted in Booth, *History of Osteopathy*, p. 57.

71. J. O. Hatten quoted in ibid., pp. 61-62. For a patient's narrative of Still's work in the 1880s, see the interview with George L. Compton in the *Kirksville Graphic*, March 19, 1897, reprinted in *J. Ost.* 3 (March 1897): 7-8.

72. Henry S. Bunting, "How Osteopathy Got Its First Recognition in Kirksville," *J. Ost.* 5 (1899): 473-75; Hildreth, *Lengthening Shadow*, pp. 13-15, 371.

73. Hildreth, *Lengthening Shadow*, p. 26.

74. Andrew T. Still, "Dr. Still's Department," *J. Ost.* 8 (1901): 68.


## Chapter 2: The Missouri Mecca

1. See E. R. N. Grigg, "Peripatetic Pioneer: William Smith, M.D., D. O. (1862-1912)," *J. Hist. Med.* 22 (1967): 169-79; "Dr. Wm. Smith, Pioneer at His Old Post," *O.P.* 12 (July 1907): 15-16.

2. William Smith as quoted in E. R. Booth, *History of Osteopathy and Twentieth-Century Medical Practice* (Cincinatti: The Caxton Press, 1924), p. 448.

3. Arthur G. Hildreth, *The Lengthening Shadow of Andrew Taylor Still* (Kirksville: Journal Printing, 1942), p. 31. The problem of securing sufficient material for dissection was an acute one for the remainder of the century. In 1897, for example, Smith and his assistant Clarence Rider traveled to Chicago, where they were able to obtain unclaimed bodies by paying off attendants at the Cook County morgue. When the "heist" had been discovered and the participants named, a warrant for Smith's arrest was issued. Fortunately for Still's anatomy instructor, the governor of Missouri refused to authorize his extra-

dition and the matter was subsequently dropped. See "Dr. Clarence L. Rider Took Part in Stirring Pioneer Affairs," *O.P.* 8 (November 1905): 13.

4. Henry S. Bunting, "Dr. William Smith Died of Pneumonia in Scotland Feb. 15th after Two Days Illness," *O.P.* 21 (March 1912): 1.

5. Henry S. Bunting, "The Real A. T. Still," *O.P.* 32 (December 1917): 16.

6. Andrew T. Still, *The Autobiography of Andrew Taylor Still* (Kirksville: By the author, 1908), pp. 184-85.

7. Ibid.

8. Hildreth, *Lengthening Shadow,* pp. 31-32, 194.

9. Andrew T. Still, "To Patients and Visitors," *J. Ost.* 1 (August 1894): 2.

10. Andrew T. Still, "Important to Patients," *J. Ost.* 2 (December 1895): 7; idem, "Address," *J. Ost.* 1 (May 1894): 1; idem, "A Plea for Temperance," *J. Ost.* 1 (June 1894): 1; idem, *Autobiography,* p. 276.

11. *St. Louis Globe-Democrat,* January 16, 1895, reprinted in *J. Ost.* 1 (January 1895): 8; *Des Moines Daily News,* November 10, 1895, reprinted in *J. Ost.* 2 (December 1895): 1; *Nebraska Daily Call,* November 17, 1895, reprinted in *J. Ost.* 2 (December 1895): 4; *Ottumwa* (Ia.) *Press,* n.d., reprinted in *J. Ost.* 1 (October 1894): 4; *Bethany* (Ill.) *Echo,* n.d., reprinted in *J. Ost.* 1 (February 1895): 2.

12. "Volume Three," *J. Ost.* 3 (June 1896): 4.

13. *Kirksville Graphic,* n.d., reprinted in *J. Ost.* 2 (September 1895): 2.

14. *Loyal Workman* (Ottumwa, Ia.), September 1, 1896, reprinted in *J. Ost.* 3 (October 1896): 1.

15. "A Glance Backward," *J. Ost.* 4 (1898): 367-74, 384-86.

16. "Invalids from Twenty-One States: A Patient Tells What He Saw at the Still Infirmary in Kirksville," *J. Ost.* 3 (June 1896): 6; *Godey's Magazine,* October 1895, reprinted in *J. Ost.* 2 (October 1895): 3.

17. These cases were originally published in the *Kirksville Journal,* January 30, 1896, and reprinted in the *J. Ost.* 2 (February 1896): 3.

18. *Cincinnati Commercial Tribune,* September 25, 1896, reprinted in *J. Ost.* 3 (October 1896): 5. See also Hildreth, *Lengthening Shadow,* pp. 85, 129; Booth, *History of Osteopathy,* pp. 46, 99. The Foraker child died at the age of thirty-nine. See "Death of A. St.C. Foraker Recalls Early Osteopathic History," *Forum of Osteopathy* (hereafter *Forum of Ost.*) 5 (1931): 176.

19. P. F. Greenwood, "The Position Osteopathy Occupies under the Present State Law," *J. Ost.* 1 (May 1894): 2.

20. "A Petition," *J. Ost.* 1 (May 1894): 4.

21. Greenwood, "Position Osteopathy Occupies," p. 2.

22. A. J. Steele, "The Osteopathic Fad," *Transactions of the Medical Association of the State of Missouri* (1895): 363.

23. "Sequel to 'The Osteopathic Fad,'" *J. Ost.* 3 (October 1896): 7.

24. William Smith, "Four Years Ago," *J. Ost.* 3 (September 1896): 6.

25. Steele, "Osteopathic Fad," p. 356.

26. E. C. Pickler and C. M. T. Hulett quoted in Booth, *History of Osteopathy,* pp. 75, 493.

27. Excerpts from the first charter can be found in the newspaper article reprinted in Hildreth, *Lengthening Shadow,* p. 34. See also Minutes of the Board of Trustees of the American School of Osteopathy, 1892, mimeographed, American Osteopathic Association Archives, Chicago.

28. Andrew T. Still, "Editorial," *J. Ost.* 3 (December 1896): 4.

29. See Booth, *History of Osteopathy,* p. 85.

30. "Legislative," *J. Ost.* 3 (February 1897): 4; "Missouri in Line," *J. Ost.* 3 (March 1897): 1.

31. "Missouri in Line," p. 1.

32. Ibid.

33. According to figures cited by E. M. Violette, the number of graduates per year jumped from 48 in 1897, to 136 in 1898, 185 in 1899, and 317 in 1900. See his *History of Adair County* (Kirksville: Journal Printing, 1911), p. 264.

34. This is most evident by the books they wrote which were among the first texts of the school. See William Smith, *Notes on Anatomy* (Kirksville: By the author, 1898); Carl P. McConnell, *Notes on Osteopathic Therapeutics* (Kirksville: By the author, 1898); Charles Hazzard, *Principles of Osteopathy*, 3d ed. (Kirksville: Journal Printing, 1899); C. W. Proctor, *A Brief Course in General Chemistry* (Kirksville: By the author, 1898); idem, *A Brief Course in Physiological Chemistry* (Kirksville: By the author, 1898); and J. Martin Littlejohn, *Physiology: Exhaustive and Practical*, 2 vols. (Kirksville: Journal Printing, 1898).

35. See Richard J. Cyriax, "A Short History of Mechano-Therapeutics in Europe until the Time of Ling," *Janus* 19 (1914): 178-88; as quoted, p. 183; pp. 189-204; as quoted, p. 225.

36. William Balfour, *Illustrations of the Power of Compression and Percussion in the Cure of Rheumatism, Gout, and Debility of the Extremities in Promoting Health and Longevity* (Edinburgh: P. Hill, 1819); John Bacot, *Observations on the Use and Abuse of Friction with Some Remarks on Motion and Rest, as Applicable to the Cure of Various Surgical Diseases* (London: Callow and Wilson, 1822); W. Cleobury, *A Full Account of the System of Friction as Adopted by J. Grosvenor and Pursued with the Greatest Success in Cases of Contracted Joints and Lameness from Various Causes* (Oxford: Munday and Slatter, 1825); S. Weir Mitchell, *Injuries of Nerves and Their Consequences* (Philadelphia: J. B. Lippincott, 1872); idem, *Fat and Blood: An Essay on the Treatment of Certain Forms of Neurasthenia and Hysteria*, 8th ed. (Philadelphia: J. B. Lippincott, 1900). Mitchell noted, "It is many years since I first saw in this city general massage used by a charlatan in a case of progressive paralysis. The temporary results he obtained were so remarkable that I began soon after to employ it in locomotor ataxia, in which it sometimes proved of signal value, and in other forms of spinal and local disease" (*Fat and Blood*, p. 81).

37. William Murrell, *Massage as a Mode of Treatment* (Philadelphia: P. Blakiston, Son, 1886), pp. 38-40; C. L. Pardington, "Massage in Migraines," *Practitioner* 37 (1886): 435-38; A. J. Eccles, "Massage as a Means of Treatment in Dyspepsia and Sleeplessness," *British Medical Journal* 2 (1877): 502-4.

38. Douglas Graham, *A Practical Treatise on Massage: Its History, Mode of Application, and Effects* (New York: William Wood, 1884).

39. George H. Taylor, *Massage: Principles and Practice of Remedial Treatment by Imparted Motion* (New York: Fowler and Wells, 1884), p. 28.

40. Graham, *Practical Treatise on Massage*, p. 35.

41. See Edgar F. Cyriax, "Concerning the Early Literature on Ling's *Medical Gymnastics*," *Janus* 30 (1926): 225-32; idem, *Bibliographia Gymnastica Medica* (n.p., 1909).

42. Hazzard, *Principles of Osteopathy*, p. 292.

43. See Murrell, *Massage as Mode of Treatment*, pp. 20-28.

44. See Francis Schiller, "Spinal Irritation and Osteopathy," *Bull. Hist. Med.* 45 (1971): 252-54.

45. See in particular Evans Riadore, *A Treatise on the Irritation of the Spinal Nerves as the Source of Nervousness, Indigestion, Functional and Organic Derangements of the Principal Organs of the Body, and on the Modifying Influence of Temperment and Habits of Man over Diseases and Their Importance as Regards Conducting Successfully the Treatment of the Latter; and on the Therapeutic Use of Water* (London: J. Churchill, 1843); and William Griffin and David Griffin, *Observations on the Functional Affections of the Spinal Cord and Ganglionic System of Nerves in which Their Identity with Sympathetic, Nervous and Irritative Diseases is Illustrated* (London: Burgess and Hill, 1844). For

additional book and article citations on the subject, see U.S. Office of the Surgeon-General, *Index-Catalogue of the Library of the U.S. Surgeon-General's Office,* 2d ser. (Washington: U.S. Government Printing Office, 1896), 13:441-43.

46. John Hilton, *On Rest and Pain: A Course of Lectures on the Influence of Mechanical and Physiological Rest on the Treatment of Accidents and Surgical Diseases, and the Diagnostic Value of Pain,* 2d ed. (New York: W. Wood, 1879).

47. Francis Schiller, noting the considerable number of works published on the subject of spinal irritation during the second and third quarters of the nineteenth century, has suggested that Still could hardly have been unaware of this doctrine. Schiller, however, was unable to marshall any hard evidence that spinal irritation had a direct influence upon Still's theory, nor have I subsequently been able to uncover any new information that would show an incontrovertible link between them. See Schiller, "Spinal Irritation and Osteopathy," pp. 250-66.

48. Hazzard, *Principles of Osteopathy,* pp. 8-13; J. Martin Littlejohn, *Principles of Osteopathy* (Chicago: By the author, 1902), pp. 2-8.

49. Walter Riese, *A History of Neurology* (New York: M. D. Publications, 1959), pp. 131-36. See also J. M. D. Olmstead, *Charles-Edouard Brown-Sequard: A Nineteenth-Century Neurologist and Endocrinologist* (Baltimore: The Johns Hopkins University Press, 1946).

50. Hazzard, *Principles of Osteopathy,* pp. 35-51.

51. Harriette Chick, Margaret Hume, and Marjorie MacFarlane, *War on Disease: A History of the Lister Institute* (London: Andre Deutsch, 1971), p. 20.

52. Andrew T. Still, "Smallpox," *Bulletin of the Atlas and Axis Clubs,* no. 3 (1901): pp. 6-7.

53. See James Littlejohn, "Bacteriology: Its History and Relation to Disease," *J. Ost.* 5 (1898): 130-34; David Littlejohn, "Diseases of a Pathogenic Origin: Indications for Treatment from an Osteopathic Standpoint," *J. Ost.* 5 (1898): 177-80; and Carl P. McConnell, *The Practice of Osteopathy* (Chicago: The Hammond Press, 1899).

54. For example, see Andrew T. Still, *Philosophy of Osteopathy* (Kirksville: By the author, 1899), p. 12.


### Chapter 3: In the Field

1. "Graduates of the American School of Osteopathy," *J. Ost.* 7 (1900): 244-48.

2. Andrew T. Still, "Dr. Still's Department," *J. Ost.* 8 (1901): 68.

3. "What is the Science of Osteopathy?" *Cosmopolitan Osteopath* 1 (November 1898): 10.

4. Therese Cluett, "The Amusing Side of Osteopathy," *Boston Osteopath* 3 (May 1900): 90.

5. Herbert Bernard quoted in E. R. Booth, *History of Osteopathy and Twentieth-Century Medical Practice* (Cincinnati: The Caxton Press, 1924), p. 60.

6. "Why Should I Try Osteopathy?" *Southern Journal of Osteopathy* 1 (November 1898): 325.

7. "Notice to Our Patrons," *Northern Osteopath* 1 (March 1897): 6.

8. "Diseases Successfully Treated by Osteopathy," *Pennsylvania Journal of Osteopathy* 1 (June 1899): 24.

9. "Diseases Treated," *New York Osteopath* 1 (April 1898): 47.

10. "Testimonials: Why We Run Them," *Osteopathic Success* 1 (February 1901): 16.

11. "Miscellaneous Cases Reported from the Field," *Popular Osteopath* 1 (1899): 156.

12. W. L. Riggs, "Osteopathy in Acute Diseases," *Cosmopolitan Osteopath* 2 (July 1899): 23.

13. A. L. Evans, "Quick Cures," *Popular Osteopath* 1 (1899): 150-51.

14. Cluett, "Amusing Side of Osteopathy," p. 90.

15. "Letters from Graduates," *J. Ost.* 4 (1898): 444.

16. Philadelphia College and Infirmary of Osteopathy, *Annual Announcement* (1899), p. 16.

17. A. L. Evans, "Why Osteopathy Is Popular," *Popular Osteopath* 1 (January 1899): 15.

18. See also "Is Osteopathy Dying Out? Have We Passed Our Zenith?" *O.P.* 14 (Nov. 1908): 1.

19. See Booth, *History of Osteopathy,* pp. 170-71; Charles E. Still, "Establishing the Fact that Osteopathy Is a Science," *J. Ost.* 4 (1898): 415-18.

20. "The Man Who Took Osteopathy to the Pacific," *O.P.* 8 (June 1905): 13.

21. Booth, *History of Osteopathy,* pp. 179-80, 181-83.

22. Ibid., p. 193.

23. See discussion ibid., pp. 162-201.

24. Ibid., pp. 191-92.

25. Ibid., pp. 106-7; Arthur G. Hildreth, *The Lengthening Shadow of Andrew Taylor Still* (Kirksville: Journal Printing, 1942), p. 94.

26. As reprinted in W. Livingston Harlan, *Osteopathy: The New Science* (Chicago: By the author, 1898), pp. 58-59.

27. "North Dakota Grit," *J. Ost.* 3 (February 1897): 1-2.

28. See Booth, *History of Osteopathy,* pp. 95-161.

29. Ibid., p. 163.

30. For a history of this process see William G. Rothstein, *American Physicians in the Nineteenth Century: From Sects to Science* (Baltimore: The Johns Hopkins University Press, 1972), pp. 298-326; Martin Kaufman, *Homeopathy in America: The Rise and Fall of a Medical Heresy* (Baltimore: The Johns Hopkins University Press, 1972), pp. 141-73.

31. These estimates are based on an examination of early alumni lists published by the colleges as well as statistics cited in Booth, *History of Osteopathy,* pp. 71-94.

32. Ibid., p. 87.

33. See, for example, the advertisement for the American College of Osteopathic Medicine and Surgery on the back cover of the *Journal of the Science of Osteopathy* (hereafter *J. Sci. Ost.*) 1 (December 1900).

34. For a contemporary critique of osteopathic colleges see C. M. Turner Hulett, "The Profession and the Schools," *J. Sci. Ost.* 1 (June 1900): 141-44.

35. "Osteopathy as a Profession," *Cosmopolitan Osteopath* 1 (July 1898): 34.

36. Mason W. Pressly, "Osteopathy as a Business," *Northern Osteopath* 2 (May 1898): 7-8.

37. "The Advantages of Osteopathy as a Study and a Profession," *Philadelphia Journal of Osteopathy* 1 (January 1899): 13.

38. "The Atlantic School of Osteopathy," *Pennsylvania Journal of Osteopathy* 1 (June 1899): 23.

39. "The Science of Osteopathy," *The Osteopath* 1 (February 1897): 4.

40. This estimate is based upon available early alumni records of several of the colleges. Of 765 total graduates listed by the American School of Osteopathy in 1900, for example, 183 (23.9 percent) were women. See "Graduates of the American School of Osteopathy," pp. 244-48.

41. Lawrence B. Finn, "The Location of the Southern School and Infirmary," *Southern Journal of Osteopathy* 1 (February 1898): 13.

42. "Editorial," *The Osteopath* 2 (August 1898): 13-14.

43. "Advantages of Des Moines—Disadvantages of Kirksville," *Cosmopolitan Osteopath* 1 (August 1898): 36-37.

44. Elmer Barber, *Osteopathy: The New Science of Healing* (Kansas City: Hudson-Kimberly Publishing, 1896). Also see his *Osteopathy Complete* (Kansas City: Hudson-Kimberly Publishing, 1898).

45. When Smith temporarily left the American School of Osteopathy for private practice after completion of the first class, his teaching duties were taken over by Nettie Bolles (died 1930), one of his students who had previously earned two bachelor's degrees. The third class in anatomy was conducted by Summerfield Still (1851-1931), the founder's nephew. Each was to found a school; the former established the Bolles Institute of Osteopathy in Denver, the latter set up the S. S. Still College of Osteopathy in Des Moines.

46. For details of the Kansas City case, see Booth, *History of Osteopathy,* pp. 86-87, 166-67.

47. See E. M. Violette, *History of Adair County* (Kirksville: Journal Printing, 1911), pp. 274-75.

48. For details see "Columbian School of Osteopathy, Medicine and Surgery," *Columbian Osteopath* 2 (October 1899): 263, 265; Violette, *History of Adair County,* p. 275.

49. J. R. Musick, "Is Osteopathy of Greek Origin?" *J. Ost.* 5 (1898): 221-25.

50. Andrew T. Still, "Dr. Still's Department," *J. Ost.* 5 (1898): 167; idem, "Medical Osteopathy," *J. Ost.* 8 (1901): 166.

51. "Cofounder of First Osteopathic College Dies," *Western Osteopath* 23 (1929): 19.

## Chapter 4: Structure and Function

1. C.M. Turner Hulett, "Historical Sketch of the A.A.A.O.," *Journal of the American Osteopathic Association* (hereafter *JAOA*) 1 (1901): 1-6; "Proceedings of the Fifth Annual Meeting of the American Association for the Advancement of Osteopathy," *JAOA* 1 (1901): 6-15.

2. "Constitution of the American Osteopathic Association," *JAOA* 1 (1901): 16-17.

3. "Constitution and By-Laws," *JAOA* 9 (1909): 37-43. See also "Should the By-Laws Be Changed?" *JAOA* 11 (1911): 667-71.

4. "Preliminary Report of the A.O.A. Committee on By-Laws," *JAOA* 18 (1919): 304-8; W. A. Gravett, "The New A.O.A.," *JAOA* 19 (1920): 191-93.

5. E. R. Booth, *History of Osteopathy and Twentieth-Century Medical Practice* (Cincinnati: The Caxton Press, 1924), pp. 106-8; A. L. Evans, "Legal Status of Osteopathy in the Various States," *JAOA* 2 (1903): 145-47.

6. Chester C. Cole, "Iowa's Medical Board and Osteopathy Law," *Cosmopolitan Osteopath* 2 (March 1899): 3-4; "Osteopathic Victory in Iowa," *JAOA* 1 (1902): 162-63.

7. See A. G. Hildreth, "Report of the Committee on Legislation with Bill Appended," *JAOA* 5 (1905): 71-75; idem, "Osteopathic Legislation," *JAOA* 2 (1903): 143-44.

8. See discussion in William G. Rothstein, *American Physicians in the Nineteenth Century: From Sects to Science* (Baltimore: The Johns Hopkins University Press, 1972), pp. 305-10.

9. A. G. Hildreth, "Osteopathic Legislation," *JAOA* 4 (1905): 191.

10. American Osteopathic Association, *Yearbook and Directory* (Chicago, 1913), pp. 97-108; American Osteopathic Association, *Yearbook and Directory* (Chicago, 1923), pp. 169-89.

11. Hulett, "Historical Sketch of the A.A.A.O.," p. 2.

12. Booth, *History of Osteopathy,* pp. 272-77.

13. "Constitution of the American Osteopathic Association," p. 16.

14. Wilfred Harris, "The Three Year Course: Some Questions for the Profession to Decide," *JAOA* 3 (1904): 373.

15. "Report of the A.O.A. Committee on Education," *JAOA* 2 (1902): 10-19.

16. C. M. Turner Hulett, "The Profession and the Schools," *J. Sci. Ost.* 1 (June 1900): 144.

17. Martin Littlejohn, "The Standard of Education," *JAOA* 1 (1902): 191-93.

18. Eamons R. Booth, "Report of Inspector of Osteopathic Schools," *JAOA* 3 (1903) supplement: 9-20.

19. "Proceedings of the Eighth Annual Meeting of the American Osteopathic Association," *JAOA* 4 (1904): 38, 51.

20. Philadelphia College and Infirmary of Osteopathy and the Osteopathic Hospital of Philadelphia, *Annual Announcement* (1919), p. 11.

21. Chicago College of Osteopathy, *Annual Catalog* (1913), pp. 15-16.

22. "Proceedings of the Philadelphia Meeting," *JAOA* 13 (1914): 727.

23. Henry S. Bunting, "Let Us Discuss Our Failures with Each Other," *O.P.* (July 1902): 1-2.

24. "Case Reports," *JAOA* 4 (1904): 96-98, 100-101.

25. A textbook based heavily upon these supplements was later issued. See Carl P. McConnell, ed., *Clinical Osteopathy* (Chicago: A. T. Still Research Institute, 1917).

26. See Edythe Ashmore, ed., "Case Reports," *JAOA* 3 (February 1904) supplement: 1-40. In the same journal: 3 (June 1904) supplement: 1-34; 4 (March 1905) supplement: 1-36; 4 (August 1905) supplement: 1-32; 5 (July 1906) supplement: 1-40; 6 (June 1907) supplement: 1-48; 7 (September 1907) supplement: 1-45; 7 (June 1908) supplement: 1-47; 7 (August 1908) supplement: 1-48; 8 (June 1909) supplement: 1-53; 8 (July 1909) supplement: 1-48; 8 (August 1909) supplement: 1-46.

27. See Fred Bischoff and Ray G. Hulbert, "The A. T. Still Research Institute: An Historical Sketch and A Look Ahead," *JAOA* 25 (1926): 376-77.

28. See John Deason and L. G. Robb, "On the Pathways for the Bulbar Respiratory Impulses in the Spinal Cord," *American Journal of Physiology* 28 (1911): 57-63. This was the product of Deason's research conducted at the Hull Physiological Laboratory of the University of Chicago.

29. See John Deason and associates, *Research in Osteopathy* (Chicago: A. T. Still Research Institute, 1916).

30. Barbara Peterson, "Louisa Burns, D.O.: Pioneer Researcher," *The D.O.* 18 (July 1978): 21-22.

31. A summary of her work is to be found in Louisa Burns and associates, *Pathogenesis of Visceral Disease following Vertebral Lesions* (Chicago: American Osteopathic Association, 1948).

32. W. V. Cole, "Louisa Burns Memorial Lecture," *JAOA* 69 (1970): 1005-17.

33. "Improper Advertising," *JAOA* 2 (1902): 85-86; *JAOA* 3 (1903): 58-59.

34. "Code of Ethics of the American Osteopathic Association," *JAOA* 4 (1904): 92-96; 95.

35. "Osteopaths Frame Code of Ethics," *O.P.* 3 (December 1902): 1-2.

36. "Code of Ethics of the American Osteopathic Association," p. 95.

37. "Report of the Committee on Education to the Board of Trustees of the American Osteopathic Association," *JAOA* 7 (1907): 87.

38. Henry S. Bunting, *The Elementary Laws of Advertising* (Chicago: The Novelty News Press, 1914).

39. Data derived from American Osteopathic Association, *Yearbook and Directory* (Chicago, 1918); American Osteopathic Association, *Yearbook and Directory* (Chicago, 1930).

40. "Hard to Distinguish Wolves When They Break into the Fold," *O.P.* 2 (July 1902): 1; "What We Do to Fakers in New York," *O.P.* 5 (May 1904): 12.

41. S. C. Matthews, "The Fake Osteopath," *The American Osteopath* 2 (September 1900): 9. See also Joseph Sullivan, "Retrospective," *The American Osteopath* 1 (June 1900): 216; W. L. Riggs, "Opposition to the Growth of Osteopathy," *Cosmopolitan Osteopath* 3 (September 1899): 3.

42. C. M. Turner Hulett, "Correspondence Schools," *JAOA* 1 (1902): 149.

43. "Report of the Committee on Education to the Board of Trustees of the American Osteopathic Association," *JAOA* 7 (1907): 87.

44. Chittenden Turner, *The Rise of Chiropractic* (Los Angeles: Powell Publishing, 1931), pp. 11-16.

45. Ibid., pp. 26-34; Ralph Lee Smith, *At Your Own Risk: The Case against Chiropractic* (New York: Trident Press, 1969), pp. 1-13.

46. Smith, *At Your Own Risk,* pp. 8-11; Turner, *Rise of Chiropractic,* pp. 35-45.

47. Edythe Ashmore, "An Imitation and Its Lessons," *JAOA* 7 (1908): 209-11, 310-11.

48. Turner, *Rise of Chiropractic,* pp. 95, 294.

## Chapter 5: Expanding the Scope

1. Minutes of the Board of Trustees of the American School of Osteopathy, 1892; mimeographed, American Osteopathic Association Archives, Chicago.

2. Andrew T. Still, "Dr. Still's Department," *J. Ost.* 8 (1901): 67.

3. Completed American Osteopathic Association School Questionnaires for the academic year 1903-4, microfilmed, American Osteopathic Association Archives, Chicago.

4. Data derived from American School of Osteopathy, *Annual Catalog* (Kirksville, 1908), pp. 24-26; American School of Osteopathy, *Annual Catalog* (Kirksville, 1918), pp. 66-68; Los Angeles College of Osteopathy, *Annual Catalog* (1908), p. 30; College of Osteopathic Physicians and Surgeons, *Annual Catalog* (Los Angeles, 1918), pp. 17-18; Philadelphia College and Infirmary of Osteopathy and the Osteopathic Hospital of Philadelphia, *Annual Announcement* (1918), pp. 21-25; Littlejohn College and Hospital, *Bulletin and Journal of Health, Announcement Number* (Chicago, 1909), p. 15; Chicago College of Osteopathy, *Annual Catalog* (1918), p. 19.

5. See Raymond S. Ward, "Why Some Osteopaths Study at Medical Colleges," *O.P.* 31 (January 1917): 25-27.

6. D. V. Morre, "Obstetrics and the General Practitioner," *JAOA* 16 (1917): 1197-98.

7. Central College of Osteopathy, *Annual Announcement* (Kansas City, 1906), p. 16.

8. Lillian M. Whiting, "Can the Length of Labor Be Shortened by Osteopathic Treatment?" *JAOA* 11 (1912): 917-21.

9. Harry L. Collins, "Origin and Progress of Osteopathic Surgery," *JAOA* 23 (1924): 715-16.

10. George A. Still, "Advantages and Necessity of Osteopathic Post-Operative Treatment," *JAOA* 18 (1919): 485.

11. See Frank P. Young, *Surgery from an Osteopathic Standpoint* (Kirksville: Journal Printing, 1904); S. L. Taylor, "Borderline Cases between Surgery and Osteopathy," *JAOA* 12 (1912): 148-54; James B. Littlejohn, "Indications for Surgical Interference in Gynecological Cases," *JAOA* 12 (1913): 331-36; "Dr. George A. Still Calls Case Reports the Profession's Most Vital Problem," *O.P.* 24 (November 1913): 3-5.

12. [Andrew T. Still], "Our Platform," *J. Ost.* 9 (October 1902): 342, later reprinted in Andrew T. Still, *Osteopathy: Research and Practice* (Kirksville: By the author, 1910), pp. 4-5.

13. Dain Tasker, "The 'Lesion' Osteopath is Too Narrow," *O.P.* 3 (January 1903): 3.

14. "'Lesions' and 'Adjuncts': The Discussion Which Occurred at Cleveland on This Subject," *JAOA* 3 (1904): 280, 283.

15. Ibid., pp. 285, 288.

16. Carl P. McConnell, *The Practice of Osteopathy* (Chicago: The Hammond Press, 1899); idem, "A Few Thoughts for the Osteopathic Practitioner," *J. Ost.* (January 1901): 9.

17. See C. W. Young, "Digest of Answers to Twelve Questions," *JAOA* 8 (1909): 358-60, 435-38. This was a survey of 260 D.O.'s on the subjects of diet, water, and "thought direction," as well as how broad osteopathy should be.

18. William G. Rothstein, *American Physicians in the Nineteenth Century: From Sects to Science* (Baltimore: The Johns Hopkins University Press, 1972), pp. 177-97.

19. See Merck and Co., *Manual of Therapeutics and Materia Medica: A Source of Ready Reference for the Physician* (Rahway, New Jersey, 1899).

20. See Hubert A. Lechevalier and Morris Solotorovsky, *Three Centuries of Microbiology* (New York: Dover Books, 1974).

21. In a commentary upon the smallpox vaccination, Still declared, "I would not antagonize the popular belief in the efficacy of vaccination but do most emphatically combat the insertion into the human body of putrid flesh of any animal" (Still, *Osteopathy: Research and Practice,* p. 456).

22. Ibid., pp. 300-301, 433-35, 470-72.

23. [Still], "Our Platform," p. 342. There was one exception, however. Still believed that a periodic application of a cantharidin blister to the arm would serve as a safer and more effective preventitive against smallpox than vaccination: "My theory is, that the first active occupant of the body by an infectious fever will drive off others and hold possession of the body until its power is spent" (Andrew T. Still, "Smallpox: Cantharidin as a Germafuge," *J. Ost.* 9 [February 1902]: 69).

24. [Andrew T. Still], "What Will Become of the M.D. D.O.?" *J. Ost.* 10 (November 1903): 366.

25. W. A. Hinckle, "A Protest against Intellectual Tyranny," *O.P.* 7 (March 1905): 11-12.

26. Some D.O.'s denied the validity of such studies. Said Riley D. Moore, "We as a profession have a few who, trusting blindly in claims made by medical authors and not knowing that medical statistics can be juggled to prove anything profitable, believe in such practice [vaccination]. But it seems to me that those who do have failed to grasp the proper conception of osteopathic principles" (Riley D. Moore, "Vaccination: Osteopaths Ought to Read up on It," *O.P.* 13 [January 1908]: 4).

27. "Correspondence," *JAOA* 8 (1908): 90-91.

28. Charles C. Teall, "Report of the Inspector of Schools," *JAOA* 6 (October 1906) supplement: 18-25.

29. E.S. Comstock, "The Littlejohn College Idea," *JAOA* 11 (1911): 675-76; "A Letter from Dr. Littlejohn," *JAOA* 11 (1911): 727-29.

30. A. B. Shaw, "The California Law and Its Workings," *JAOA* 13 (1914): 283-84; "Report of the Committee on Education," *JAOA* 12 (1913): 746-47; Dain Tasker, "Notes on Medical Legislation in California," *JAOA* 15 (1916): 398-404.

31. Teall, "Report of the Inspector," pp. 19-20.

32. Des Moines Still College of Osteopathy, *Annual Catalog* (1908), p. 50.

33. American School of Osteopathy, *Annual Catalog* (Kirksville, 1911), p. 35.

34. "The Message from Philadelphia," *JAOA* 13 (1914): 720-24.

35. "New Legislation in Oregon Causes Dissension," *O.P.* 26 (March 1915): 8-9.

36. Henry S. Bunting, "What is *Meteria Medica* Anyway? How Far Are We against It?" *O.P.* 27 (June 1915): 5-6.

37. "Sentiment in Oregon Divided on New Law,"*O.P.* 28 (July 1915): 9.

38. As reprinted in E. R. Booth, *History of Osteopathy and Twentieth-Century Medical Practice* (Cincinnati: The Caxton Press, 1924), p. 442.

39. "Espousing Academic Freedom Was the Most Notable Work of the Portland Convention," *O.P.* 28 (August 1915): 1-3.

40. Alfred W. Crosby, Jr., *Epidemic and Peace* (Westport: Greenwood Press, 1976),

pp. 206-7. See also A. A. Hoehling, *The Great Epidemic* (Boston: Little, Brown, 1961).

41. William Osler, *Principles and Practice of Medicine*, 8th ed. (New York: D. Appleton, 1912), p. 119.

42. Carl P. McConnell, "Editorial: The Treatment of Influenza," *JAOA* 18 (1918): 83-85; C. C. Reed, "Prevention and Treatment of Influenza," *JAOA* 18 (1919): 209-11; L. K. Tuttle and Robert W. Rogers, "Influenza and Pneumonia Treatment," *JAOA* 18 (1919): 211-14; George M. McCole, "Spanish or Epidemic Influenza from the Treatment Side," *O.P.* 35 (June 1919): 1-6.

43. "Osteopathy's Epidemic Record," *O.P.* 36 (July 1919): 1; "Death Statistics Reveal Comparative Values of Osteopath and Drug Treatments," *O.P.* 34 (December 1918): 1-2.

44. "Editorial: Figures Never Lie," *JAMA* 72 (1919): 731.

45. "The Profession's Policy," *JAOA* 19 (1920): 482-83; "Report of the Associated Colleges," *JAOA* 19 (1920) supplement: 6-7.

46. As of 1927 only eleven states gave D.O.'s the same unlimited license privileges granted to M.D.'s. See American Osteopathic Association, *Digest of State Laws Relating to Osteopathy* (Chicago, 1927).

47. E. S. Comstock, "A Professional Problem," *JAOA* 23 (1924): 524; idem, "Chicago College Curriculum," *JAOA* 24 (1925): 460; Asa Willard, "*Materia Medica* in the Colleges," *JAOA* 25 (1925): 279.

48. George H. Carpenter, "Between the Devil and the Deep Blue Sea, or Damned If We Do and Damned If We Don't," *Forum of Ost.* 2 (December 1928): 3-4.

49. "Proceedings of the House of Delegates," *Forum of Ost.* 3 (August 1929) supplement: 5.

50. "Correspondence: *Materia Medica,*" *Forum of Ost.* 2 (October 1928): 14-15; *Forum of Ost.* 2 (November 1928): 10-11; H. L. Knapp, "An Open Letter to Dr. John A. MacDonald," *Forum of Ost.* 2 (December 1928): 3; Warren B. Davis, "People Want Osteopathy," *Forum of Ost.* 2 (February 1929): 7.

51. "Proceedings of the House of Delegates," *Forum of Ost.* 3 (August 1929) supplement: 6.

52. "Proceedings of the House of Delegates," *Forum of Ost.* 4 (October 1930) supplement: 6-8.

## Chapter 6: The Push for Higher Standards

1. William G. Rothstein, *American Physicians in the Nineteenth Century: From Sects to Science* (Baltimore: The Johns Hopkins University Press, 1972), pp. 309-10.

2. John Field, "Medical Education in the United States: Late Nineteenth and Twentieth Centuries," in *The History of Medical Education*, ed. C. D. O'Malley (Berkeley and Los Angeles: University of California Press, 1970), pp. 508-9. See also V. Johnson and H. G. Weiskotten, *A History of the Council on Medical Education and Hospitals of the American Medical Association* (Chicago: American Medical Association, 1960).

3. Abraham Flexner, *Medical Education in the United States and Canada: A Report to the Carnegie Foundation for the Advancement of Teaching* (Boston: The Merrymount Press, 1910), pp. 62-67, 91-103.

4. Ibid., p. 151.

5. Carelton B. Chapman, "The Flexner Report," *Daedalus* 103 (Winter 1974): 110-12.

6. There were ninety-five M.D.-granting schools in the United States in 1915; eighty-five in 1920; and seventy-one in 1927. See Morris Fishbein, *A History of the American Medical Association, 1847 to 1947* (Philadelphia: W. B. Saunders, 1947), p. 898.

7. H. G. Weiskotten et al., *Medical Education in the United States, 1934-1939* (Chicago: American Medical Association, 1940), p. 15.

8. Ibid., pp. 67, 107.

9. Saul Jarcho, "Medical Education in the United States, 1910-1956," *Journal of the*

*Mt. Sinai School of Medicine* 26 (1957): 351; Field, "Medical Education," pp. 512-13.

10. Of the 5,611 M.D.'s graduating in 1935, 5,491 (97.8 percent) immediately entered approved internships. See "Medical Education in the United States and Canada: Data for the Academic Year 1935-36," *JAMA* 107 (1936): 669.

11. Flexner, *Medical Education,* p. 164.

12. Ibid., pp. 164-66.

13. Ibid., p. 166.

14. "Carnegie Foundation Report," *JAOA* 10 (1911): 621-22.

15. "Report of the Committee on Education," *JAOA* 10 (1910): 35-38.

16. John E. Rogers, "Report of the Committee on College Instruction," *JAOA* 31 (1932): 509; Completed AOA Survey Questionnaire of Osteopathic Colleges for the academic year 1931-32, microfilmed, American Osteopathic Association Archives, Chicago.

17. George A. Laughlin, "Hindrances to Osteopathic Progress," *JAOA* 24 (1925): 519. Upon Still's death in 1917 his grandnephew George A. Still became president. A family struggle ensued, resulting in some members leaving the American School of Osteopathy. In 1922 Laughlin, an orthopedic surgeon, opened a rival school in Kirksville, The Andrew Taylor Still College of Osteopathy and Surgery. Upon George Still's death that same year, negotiations were begun for the merger of the two institutions, which was effected in 1924. See. E. R. Booth, *History of Osteopathy and Twentieth-Century Medical Practice* (Cincinnati: The Caxton Press, 1924), pp. 548-49.

18. Laughlin, "Hindrances to Osteopathic Progress," p. 519.

19. R. H. Singleton, "Report of Committee on American Osteopathic Foundation," *JAOA* 31 (1932): 511. See also John E. Rogers, "Report of the Bureau of Professional Education and Colleges," *JAOA* 36 (1937): 607.

20. See Asa Willard, "State Legal and Legislative Matters," *Forum of Ost.* 4 (October 1930) supplement: 12.

21. This school is not to be confused with the Central College of Osteopathy, also of Kansas City.

22. Ira W. Drew and Edgar O. Holden, "A Brief Sketch of the History of the Philadelphia College of Osteopathy with a View to the Future," *Osteopathic Digest* 20 (January 1950): 50-51.

23. For example, see A. W. Bailey, "Osteopathic Education," *JAOA* 24 (1925): 355-58.

24. "Medical Education in the United States and Canada: Data for the Academic Year 1935-36," pp. 684-85.

25. Data derived from AOA Completed Survey Questionnaires of Osteopathic Colleges for the academic year 1935-36, microfilmed, American Osteopathic Association Archives, Chicago.

26. Data derived from college catalogs.

27. College of Osteopathic Physicians and Surgeons, *Annual Announcement* (Los Angeles, 1935), p. 71.

28. See John P. Wood, "Public Tax Supported Hospitals," *JAOA* 50 (1951): 141-44.

29. George W. Woodbury, "Unit Number Two of the Los Angeles County General Hospital: What It Is and How It Came About," *Western Osteopath* 23 (September 1928): 7-11.

30. Precisely how many osteopathic hospitals there were in this period is not known, since such institutions were under no obligation to identify themselves to the AOA. See Edgar O. Holden, "Report of the Bureau of Hospitals," *JAOA* 35 (1935): 46.

31. John E. Rogers, "Report of Bureau of Professional Education and Colleges," *JAOA* (1932): 508.

32. As derived from American Osteopathic Association, *Abstract of Laws Governing the Practice of Osteopathy* (Chicago, 1937), pp. 3-15.

33. Osteopathic data from "Report of the American Association of Osteopathic Examiners: 1952," microfilmed, American Osteopathic Association Archives, Chicago; M.D. data derived from "Medical Education in the United States," *JAMA* 90 (1928): 1203; *JAMA* 92 (1929): 1434-35; *JAMA* 94 (1930): 1312-13; *JAMA* 96 (1931): 1392-93; *JAMA* 98 (1932): 1460-61.

34. In 1907, 40.5 percent of all AOA listed D.O.'s were located in five states that had colleges: California, Illinois, Iowa, Missouri, and Pennsylvania. In 1940 this figure stood at 42.1 percent. Data derived from American Osteopathic Association, *Yearbook and Directory* (Chicago, 1907); American Osteopathic Association, *Yearbook and Directory* (Chicago, 1940).

35. See Robert G. Derbyshire, *Medical Licensure and Discipline in the United States* (Baltimore: The Johns Hopkins University Press, 1969), pp. 118-33.

36. As quoted in Asa Willard, "Basic Science Boards," *Forum of Ost.* 2 (November 1928): 2.

37. "State Board Statistics for 1930," *JAMA* 96 (1931): 1399.

38. Willard, "State Legal and Legislative Matters," p. 13.

39. As quoted in Willard, "Basic Science Boards," p. 3.

40. Frederick Etherinton and S. Stanley Ryerson, "Preliminary Report to the Joint Advisory Committee Representing the College of Physicians and Surgeons of Ontario, the Ontario Medical Association, and the Universities in Ontario Engaged in the Teaching of Medicine on Osteopathic Colleges and Teaching in Kirksville, Philadelphia, Des Moines, and Chicago," March 1, 1934, microfilmed, American Osteopathic Association Archives, Chicago.

41. See "Report of the Council on Medical Education and Hospitals," *JAMA* 114 (1940): 1926.

42. See Ray G. Hulburt, "The Ontario Investigation of Osteopathy," *JAOA* 34 (1935): 466-71. Although the official report of Etherington and Ryerson was straightforward and factual, other statements by them tended to support the D.O.'s' charges. See Frederick Etherington, "Osteopathy and Licensure," *JAMA* 104 (1935): 1549-52.

43. L. E. Blauch, "Studies of the Chicago, Des Moines, Kansas City and Philadelphia Osteopathic Colleges," 1936, microfilmed, American Osteopathic Association Archives, Chicago. Blauch's Kirksville study is not included in the archival collection.

44. "Entrance Requirements, Enrollments, Next Steps," *JAOA* 39 (1939): 225-26. In 1943 the AOA began enforcing a requirement that the matriculant had to have also taken a minimum number of courses in English, biology, physics, and chemistry. See R. McFarlane Tilley, "Report of the Bureau of Professional Education and Colleges," *JAOA* 43 (1943): 81-83.

45. Asa Willard, "Where Our Students Come From," *JAOA* 46 (1947): 313.

46. Lawrence Mills, "Colleges Visited," *JAOA* 45 (1946): 422; *JAOA* 46 (1947): 591-92.

47. See Lawrence Mills, "Applications to Osteopathic Colleges," *JAOA* 51 (1952): 541-42.

48. Lawrence Mills, "Osteopathic Education," *JAOA* 50 (1951): 277-78.

49. Data derived from college catalogs.

50. Data derived from abstracted minutes of the sessions of the American Association of Osteopathic Colleges, 1945-60, microfilmed, American Osteopathic Association Archives, Chicago.

51. Data derived from college catalogs.

52. Data derived from completed AOA Hospital Questionnaires for the year 1960, microfilmed, American Osteopathic Association Archives, Chicago.

53. Data derived from college catalogs.

54. "Osteopathic Progress Fund Reaches $962,535 as of June 15th," *JAOA* 43 (1944): 527.

55. Figures derived from "Recap of Annual Cash Received by the Osteopathic Progress Fund, 1946-1975," typescript, American Osteopathic Association Archives, Chicago.

56. "Cancer Teaching Grants to Osteopathic Colleges," *JAOA* 51 (1951): 126. "Six

Colleges Report USPHS Grants," *Forum of Ost.* 30 (1956): 292. "Hospital Survey and Construction Act," *JAOA* 46 (1946): 24-26; "Important Change in Hospital Construction Act Regulations," *JAOA* 46 (1947): 570.

57. See American Osteopathic Association, *Standardization of Osteopathic Hospitals Including Codes, Hospital Regulations, Requirements for Teaching of Interns,* 2d ed. (Chicago, February 1938).

58. R. C. McCaughan, "Report of the Executive Secretary," *JAOA* 45 (1945): 23.

59. Floyd F. Peckham, "Report of the Bureau of Hospitals," *JAOA* 51 (1951): 74.

60. "AOA History: Dates, Events, and People," *JAOA* 77 (April 1978) supplement: 10.

61. R. McFarlane Tilley, "Report of the Advisory Board for Osteopathic Specialists," *JAOA* 39 (1939): 74-75.

62. See R. C. McCaughan, "Report of the Executive Secretary," *JAOA* 42 (1942): 46; R. McFarlane Tilley, "Report of the Bureau of Professional Education and Colleges," *JAOA* 46 (1946): 75; *JAOA* 47 (1947): 78-79; *JAOA* 49 (1949): 57; *JAOA* 50 (1950): 76. Also see Robert B. Thomas, "Report of the Bureau of Professional Education and Colleges," *JAOA* 53 (1953): 75. American Osteopathic Association, *Abstract of Laws and Regulations Governing the Practice of Osteopathy* (Chicago, 1960), p. 2.

## Chapter 7: A Question of Identity

1. Robert B. Thomas, "Report of the Council on Education," *JAOA* 50 (1950): 88.

2. G. W. Woodbury, "The Treasure of Distinctive Osteopathy," *JAOA* 39 (1940): 367.

3. E. A. Ward, "Pneumonia: Comparative Therapeutics," *JAOA* 49 (1950): 318-20; Floyd Peckham, "How to Obtain Better Cooperation between the Profession and the Hospital," *JAOA* 45 (1946): 199-200.

4. C. Robert Starks, "Our Greatest Challenge," *JAOA* 45 (1946): 537.

5. Floyd F. Peckham, "Report of the Bureau of Hospitals," *JAOA* 51 (1951): 74.

6. See Raymond P. Keesecker, "The Road Ahead for Osteopathy," *Forum of Ost.* 29 (1955): 283; Woodbury, "Treasure of Distinctive Osteopathy," p. 367; Stanley Evans, "Future of Osteopathy," *Osteopathic Profession* 15 (March 1948): 12.

7. See J. McKee Arthur, "The Editor's Page," *Osteopathic Profession* 9 (1942): 28-29.

8. Henry S. Bunting, "Finding Ourselves in This Antitoxin Problem," *O.P.* 29 (January 1916): 2-3. See also Robert H. Nichols, "Editorial: Reasonable Arguments," *Osteopathic Research Internist* 1 (December 1924): 163-66.

9. J. Steadman Denslow, "Guest Editorial: Ralph Waldo Gerard, Distinguished and Courageous Scientist," *JAOA* 73 (1974): 793-96.

10. J. Steadman Denslow and G. H. Clough, "Reflex Activity in the Spinal Extensors," *Journal of Neurophysiology* 4 (1941): 430-37; J. Steadman Denslow and C. C. Hassett, "The Central Excitatory State Associated with Postural Abnormalities," *Journal of Neurophysiology* 5 (1942): 393-402; J. Steadman Denslow and C. C. Hassett, "The Polyphasic Action Currents of the Motor Unit Complex," *American Journal of Physiology* 139 (1943): 652-59; J. Steadman Denslow, "Analysis of Variability of Spinal Reflex Thresholds," *Journal of Neurophysiology* 7 (1944): 207-15.

11. J. Steadman Denslow, Irwin M. Korr, and A. D. Krems, "Quantitative Studies of Chronic Facilitation in Human Motor Neuron Pools," *American Journal of Physiology* 105 (1947): 229-38.

12. See W. V. Cole, *An Introduction to Osteopathic Medicine* (Kansas City: Kansas City College of Osteopathy and Surgery, 1961), pp. 64-65.

13. Louis Chandler, "Physiological Integration as a Basis for Recovery from Disease and Its Osteopathic Implication," *JAOA* 49 (1950): 305-15.

14. For a more detailed summary of pharmocotherapeutic advances in this era, see Ernst

Baumler, *In Search of the Magic Bullet* (London: Thames and Hudson, 1965), and L. Earle Arnow, *Health in a Bottle* (Philadelphia: J. B. Lippincott, 1970).

15. Minutes of the AOA Board of Trustees, July 19-23, 1948, microfilmed, American Osteopathic Association Archives, Chicago, pp. 72-73.

16. In 1951 the House of Delegates passed a resolution urging the various boards of specialty certification to "insist upon a well developed understanding of osteopathic principles and a demonstrated ability to apply those principles as a primary prerequisite for certification as an osteopathic specialist." See "Proceedings of the House of Delegates," *JAOA* 51 (1951): 25.

17. Margaret W. Barnes, "A Fortieth Anniversary Memoir," *The D.O.* 18 (January 1978): 25-29; Margaret W. Barnes, "History of the Academy of Applied Osteopathy," *The D.O.* 12 (June 1972): 113-33.

18. Lawrence Mills, "Adequacy of Undergraduate Osteopathic Teaching as Judged by Osteopathic Physicians Who Graduated from 1948 through 1953," microfilmed, American Osteopathic Association Archives, Chicago.

19. Data culled from American Osteopathic Association, *Yearbook and Directory* (Chicago, 1960).

20. "The Man on the Street Gives His Ideas on Osteopathy," *Forum of Ost.* 11 (1937): 35, 51-52.

21. George W. Hartmann, "The Relative Social Prestige of Representative Medical Specialties," *Journal of Applied Psychology* 20 (1936): 659-63.

22. L. Alice Foley, "Osteopaths or Osteopathic Physicians," *JAOA* 25 (1926): 371; M. F. Hulett, "Osteopathic Physician and Surgeon," *JAOA* 25 (1926): 458; Cyrus Gaddis, "Away from Congested Centers," *JAOA* 26 (1926): 204.

23. "New Medical Dictionary Defines Osteopathy," *Forum of Ost.* 10 (1936): 205; Ray G. Hulburt, "Definitions—Spinal Joints—Osteopathic Physicians," *Forum of Ost.* 5 (1931): 194-95; George M. McCole, "Osteopathic Definitions," *Forum of Ost.* 10 (1936): 151, 168.

24. "Proceedings of the House of Delegates," *Forum of Ost.* 3 (August 1929): 6; "Osteopathic Physicians in Directories," *Forum of Ost.* 1 (December 1927): 12; R. C. McCaughan, "Report of the Executive Secretary," *JAOA* 36 (1937): 594-96.

25. "Federal Emergency Sick Relief," *Forum of Ost.* 7 (1933): 183-84; "F.E.R.A. and C.W.A.," *Forum of Ost.* 7 (1934): 263; "Where Do We Go from Here?" *Forum of Ost.* 12 (1938): 97, 114; B. F. Adams, "Report of the Committee on Compensation Insurance," *JAOA* 46 (1946): 93-94; Robert K. Homan, "Report of the Committee on Compensation Insurance," *JAOA* 48 (1948): 69; John P. Wood, "The Audrain County Hospital Case," *JAOA* 50 (1951): 292-93; Don Cameron, "Can a Hospital Survive a D.O. Invasion?" *Medical Economics* 30 (July 1953): 99-105; "Hospital Survey and Construction Act," *JAOA* 46 (1946): 24-26; "Important Change in Hospital Construction Act Regulations," *JAOA* 46 (1947): 570.

26. Mark Sullivan, "If I Need Relaxation," *Reader's Digest* 34 (February 1939): 86-88.

27. Perhaps the most publicity osteopathy has ever received came as a result of the trials of Sam Sheppard, D.O., in Ohio during the 1950s and 1960s. As one osteopathic leader ironically noted, it was through this case that thousands of Americans learned for the first time that a D.O. could be a neurosurgeon. See Jackson Harrison Pollack, *Dr. Sam: An American Tragedy* (Chicago: Henry Regnery, 1972).

28. Raymond Keesecker, "To the Student Wife," *Forum of Ost.* 29 (1955): 322-23. See also Peter K. New, "The Osteopathic Students: A Study in Dilemma," in *Patients, Physicians and Illness,* ed. E. Gartly Jaco (Glencoe: Free Press, 1958), pp. 413-21.

29. O. W. Barnes, "Fifty Years Forecast of Osteopathy," *Forum of Ost.* 3 (1929): 119; "Heresy or Science? Should We Award M.D. Degrees?" *Forum of Ost.* 9 (1935): 29-31, 38.

30. R. McFarlane Tilley, "Report of the Bureau of Professional Education and Colleges," *JAOA* 41 (1941): 58, 59.

31. Donald M. Lewis, "D.O. and M.D.," *Forum of Ost.* 1 (May 1927): 20; Abridged Proceedings, Mid-Year Meeting of the Executive Committee of the Board of Trustees, December 18-20, 1942, microfilmed, American Osteopathic Association Archives, Chicago, pp. 35, 132-33.

32. This failure to identify one's osteopathic affiliation also extended to the hospitals. However, in 1947 the AOA house mandated that all such facilities include either the word *osteopathy* or the word *osteopathic* in their title or subtitle. See Floyd F. Peckham, "Report of the Bureau of Hospitals," *JAOA* 47 (1947): 92.

### Chapter 8: The California Merger

1. See Louisa H. Bartosh, "The History of Osteopathy in California," *Journal of the Osteopathic Physicians and Surgeons of California* 5 (April/May 1978): 30-33.

2. W. Ballentine Henley, "Comes the Dawn," *JAOA* 58 (1958): 141-47.

3. "Proceedings of the House of Delegates," *JAOA* 40 (1940): 33-34.

4. For a discussion of the absorption of the homeopaths and eclectics, see William G. Rothstein, *American Physicians in the Nineteenth Century: From Sects to Science* (Baltimore: The Johns Hopkins University Press, 1972), pp. 298-326.

5. Arnold I. Kisch and Arthur J. Viseltear, *Doctors of Medicine and Doctors of Osteopathy in California: Two Medical Professions Face the Problem of Providing Medical Care* (Arlington, Va.: Department of Health, Education and Welfare, Public Health Service, Division of Medical Care Administration, 1967), pp. 14-15.

6. Minutes of the California Osteopathic Association House of Delegates and Board of Trustees, March 18-19, 1944, microfilmed, American Osteopathic Association Archives, Chicago, pp. 5-6.

7. Ibid., p. 7; Kisch and Viseltear, *Doctors of Medicine*, p. 15.

8. Minutes of the California Osteopathic Association House of Delegates and Board of Trustees, March 18-19, 1944, p. 7; Minutes of the California Osteopathic Association, Report of the Fact-Finding Committee, March 3-4, 1945, microfilmed, American Osteopathic Association Archives, Chicago.

9. Metropolitan University, College of Medicine and Surgery, Graduate Division, *Annual Catalog* (Los Angeles, 1945); Metropolitan University File, microfilmed, American Osteopathic Association Archives, Chicago.

10. Minutes of the American Osteopathic Association Board of Trustees, July 1948, microfilmed, American Osteopathic Association Archives, Chicago, pp. 171-75.

11. Kisch and Viseltear, *Doctors of Medicine*, p. 15.

12. Ibid.

13. Minutes of the American Osteopathic Association Board of Trustees, July 11-15, 1949, microfilmed, American Osteopathic Association Archives, Chicago, pp. 201-2; Minutes of the California Osteopathic Association House of Delegates and Board of Trustees, April 27-28, 1949, microfilmed, American Osteopathic Association Archives, Chicago, p. 15.

14. Facts Relating to the Origins of the AOA-AMA Conference Committee Meetings, n.d., microfilmed, American Osteopathic Association Archives, Chicago, p. 4.

15. Ibid., pp. 5-6.

16. "Editorial: The AOA and AMA Conferences," *Forum of Ost.* 27 (1953): 186-87.

17. Wire Recording Notes Taken March 8, 1952, by the American Osteopathic Association Conference Committee, microfilmed, American Osteopathic Association Archives, Chicago.

18. "Editorial: The AOA and AMA Conferences," p. 187.

19. Ibid.

20. "Address of the President, Dr. John W. Cline," *JAMA* 149 (1952): 853-56; "Report of the Reference Committee on Miscellaneous Business," *JAMA* 149 (1952): 944; "Report of Officers," *JAMA* 150 (1952): 892; "Report of the Judicial Council," *JAMA* 150 (1952): 1706.

21. "Editorial: The AOA and AMA Conferences," p. 188.

22. "Report of the Committee for the Study of Relations Between Osteopathy and Medicine," *JAMA* 152 (1953): 734-39.

23. Report of the American Osteopathic Association Conference Committee to the A.O.A. House of Delegates, July 1954, microfilmed, American Osteopathic Association Archives, Chicago, p. 2.

24. Ibid., pp. 2-7.

25. Ibid., pp. 11-17.

26. Ibid., pp. 17-19.

27. Minutes of the American Osteopathic Association House of Delegates, July 1954, microfilmed, American Osteopathic Association Archives, Chicago, p. 281.

28. "Supplementary Report of the Board of Trustees," *JAMA* 156 (1954): 1600-1605; "The ALA and AMA Conferences: To Settle with Finality," *Forum of Ost.* 28 (1954): 611-14.

29. "Report of the Committee for the Study of Relations between Osteopathy and Medicine," *JAMA* 158 (1955): 736-42.

30. Ibid., p. 740.

31. Ibid., p. 741.

32. Ibid., pp. 41-42.

33. Minutes of the Meeting of the American Osteopathic Association Conference Committee, June 11, 1955, microfilmed, American Osteopathic Association Archives, Chicago, pp. 1-5.

34. "The AOA and AMA Conferences: Settled without Finality," *Forum of Ost.* 29 (1955): 244-47.

35. True B. Eveleth to Floyd F. Peckham, November 21, 1957, microfilmed, American Osteopathic Association Archives, Chicago.

36. "Proceedings of the House of Delegates," *JAOA* 57 (1957): 68.

37. Ibid.

38. "Highlights of the Twelfth Clinical Meeting," *JAMA* 168 (1958): 2150.

39. "Report of the Judicial Council," *JAMA* 171 (1959): 978-79.

40. "Highlights of the Atlantic City Meeting," *JAMA* 170 (1959): 1075; "M.D.'s Can Teach D.O.'s—If," *American Osteopathic Association News Bulletin* (hereafter *AOA News Bull.*) (June 1959): 1-2.

41. "Remarks of George W. Northup, D.O., to the House of Delegates, July 12, 1959," microfilmed, American Osteopathic Association Archives, Chicago, pp. 1-5.

42. "Text of Michigan Resolution," *AOA News Bull.* 3 (August 1959): 1.

43. Kisch and Viseltear, *Doctors of Medicine,* pp. 23-24.

44. Ibid., pp. 25-27; "A.O.A. Acts on Unity Talks," *AOA News Bull.* 3 (August 1960): 1.

45. "Text of Michigan Resolution," p. 3.

46. Kisch and Viseltear, *Doctors of Medicine,* p. 28; "C.O.A. Charter Revoked," *AOA News Bull.* 3 (November 1960): 1.

47. "A.O.A. Charters New Group," *AOA News Bull.* 4 (February 1961): 1.

48. Kisch and Viseltear, *Doctors of Medicine,* p. 31.

49. "A Report to the Membership," *JAOA* 60 (1961): 671-74.

50. Kisch and Viseltear, *Doctors of Medicine,* pp. 34-36.

51. Ibid., pp. 33-34.

52. "California Merger Program: Important Dates," microfilmed, American Osteopathic Association Archives, Chicago.

1. "Osteopathy: Special Report of the Judicial Council to the AMA House of Delegates," *JAMA* 177 (1961): 775.

2. "Editorial: Osteopaths vs. Osteopathy," *JAMA* 177 (1961): 779.

3. "Osteopathy: Special Report of the Judicial Council," p. 775.

4. "Trustees Statement on A.M.A. Policy," *AOA News Bull.* 4 (July 1961): 3.

5. Ibid. Following this line of reasoning, economist Erwin Blackstone has recently argued that the principal motivation behind this and other AMA policies towards the D.O.'s was a desire to eliminate a viable competitor. See his "The A.M.A. and the Osteopaths: A Study of the Power of Organized Medicine," *The Antitrust Bulletin* 22 (1977): 405-40.

6. "Medical Societies Confer with Osteopaths," *AMA News* 8 (March 1, 1965): 2.

7. "Washington State M.D.-D.O. Plan Told," *AMA News* 6 (November 11, 1963): 16; "M.D.-D.O. Merger Efforts Continue," *AMA News* 7 (April 13, 1964): 16; "M.D. Degrees for Osteopaths Validated," *AMA News* 10 (January 9, 1967): 9; "Osteopaths' M.D. Degrees Denied," *AMA News* 11 (January 8, 1968): 1, 11.

8. "D.O.'s Attend Town Hall Meeting to Discuss Current A.O.A. Policies," *AOA News Bull.* 5 (May 1962): 1; "A.O.A. Will Hold Town Hall Session at M.A.O.P.S. Meeting," *AOA* News Bull. 5 (October, 1962): 1.

9. Galen Young, "Message from the President of the A.O.A.," *JAOA* 59 (1960): 487-88.

10. Arnold I. Kisch and Arthur J. Viseltear, *Doctors of Medicine and Doctors of Osteopathy in California: Two Medical Professions Face the Problem of Providing Medical Care* (Arlington, Va.: Department of Health, Education and Welfare, Public Health Service, Division of Medical Care Administration, 1967), p. 40; "When D.O.'s Become M.D.'s," *Medical Economics* 40 (December 2, 1963): 62.

11. See Nancy Kaye, "D.O.'s Turned M.D.: How Are They Faring?" *Medical Economics* 40 (November 4, 1963): 115-25.

12. Kisch and Viseltear, *Doctors of Medicine,* p. 42.

13. Ibid., p. 41.

14. "Profile of a Merger: Responses to Questionnaires, Analyses, Comments Conducted November 17-20, 1965, in California by the A.O.A. Public Relations Department," microfilmed, American Osteopathic Association Archives, Chicago.

15. Ibid., p. 6.

16. Ibid.

17. "Sues to Stop Recognition of Little m.d. by New York," *AOA News Bull.* 9 (February 1966): 5. In New York, however, as a result of an administrative decision by the State Department of Education, D.O.'s who held 1961 California College of Medicine diplomas could be listed on their license if they so chose as "D.O.-M.D.," though they were examined and licensed on the basis of their osteopathic credentials. This practice, however, was stopped by the courts in 1968, although the fifteen D.O.'s who had already opted to do so won the right to retain this designation. "Fifteen New 'D.O.-M.D.'s' Result from New York's Ruling," *AMA News* 7 (February 17, 1964): 16; "Certificate Listing 'M.D.-D.O.' Prompts New York Lawsuit," *AMA News* 9 (February 28, 1966): 9; "Osteopaths' M.D. Degrees Denied," *AMA News* 11 (January 8, 1968): 1, 11; "Osteopath Can Display 'M.D.,'" *AMA News* 13 (February 2, 1970): 14.

18. See Kaye, "D.O.'s Turned M.D.: How Are They Faring?"

19. Jack Leahy, "How D.O.'s Feel about AOA-AMA Relations," *O.P.* 38 (July 1972): 28.

20. "A.H.A. Changes Listing Criteria," *AOA News Bull.* 2 (September 1959): 1, 3.

21. "Joint Commission Okays Mixed Staffs," *AOA News Bull.* 3 (October 1960): 1.

22. "Changes in D.O. Policy Opposed," *AMA News* 8 (May 3, 1965): 7; "Medicolegal Decisions," *AMA News* 11 (November 25, 1968): 13; "Oppressive Actions in Maryland, Nebraska Seek to Deny Full Licensing of D.O.'s," *AOA News Bull.* 8 (May 1965): 3.

23. "D.O.'s Qualify for Positions with U.S. Civil Service," *AOA News Bull.* 6 (May 1963): 2; "Order Armed Forces to Commission D.O.'s as Medical Officers," *AOA News Bull.* 9 (June 1966): 1; "U.S. Recognizes A.O.A. Hospital Accreditation for Use in Medicare," *AOA News Bull.* 9 (November 1966): 1, 8.

24. "D.O. Education Changes Urged," *AMA News* 10 (July 3, 1967): 1, 8. See also "House of Delegates Meets," *JAMA* 201 (1967): 38.

25. "House of Delegates Rebuffs 'Academic Piracy' of A.M.A.," *AOA News Bull.* 10 (August 1967): 1, 8.

26. See Carl Waterbury, "D.O.-M.D.: Some Guidelines," *O.P.* 35 (November 1969): 17-19. J. Dudley Chapman, "The Other Side of the Des Moines College Crisis," *O.P.* 36 (July 1970): 17-23; "Dr. Waterbury Speaks Out on C.O.M.S.," *O.P.* 37 (May 1971): 21-23.

27. "A.M.A. Offers Means for D.O. Membership," *AMA News* 11 (December 16, 1968): 1, 8.

28. "D.O.'s Can Now Join A.M.A.," *AMA News* 12 (July 28, 1969): 6; "Eligibility of Osteopaths for County and State Medical Society Membership," *JAMA* 210 (1969): 1512.

29. "House of Delegates Takes Action to Resolve Conflict of Interest," *AOA News Bull.* 11 (August 1968): 1; "A.O.A. House of Delegates Reaffirms Separate Status for D.O.'s," *American Osteopathic Association News Review* 12 (September 1969): 1-2.

30. Edward P. Crowell, "A.O.A. House and Board Meet in Denver: Reaffirm Membership Policy, Approve Health Insurance Statement," *The D.O.* 12 (October 1971): 45-46, 56-58; idem, "A.O.A. Board and House Meet: Take Significant Actions," *The D.O.* 14 (October 1973): 75-76.

31. Data furnished by the American Medical Association, Department of Membership.

32. "Dual Membership Rare, A.O.A. Says," *AMA News* 19 (September 6, 1976): 18.

33. Data culled from American Osteopathic Association, *Yearbook and Directory* (Chicago, 1968); American Osteopathic Association, *Yearbook and Directory* (Chicago, 1978).

34. "A.O.A. House of Delegates Reaffirms Separate Status," pp. 1-2.

35. Carolyn E. Cranford, "A.O.A.-A.A.O.C. Meet in Chicago," *The D.O.* 10 (February 1970): 51.

36. Barbara Peterson, "A.O.A. House of Delegates Moves to Serve the Public Health," *The D.O.* 11 (September 1970): 53.

37. "Editorials," *JAOA* 70 (1970): 104.

38. In the year 1972 to 1973 there were 415 D.O.'s in AOA-accredited hospital residencies. In the year 1976 to 1977 the figure was 531. See American Association of Colleges of Osteopathic Medicine, *Final Report of the Osteopathic Medical Manpower Information Project* (Washington, 1977), p. 41.

39. "Osteopathy Ruling Voided," *American Medical News* 16 (October 15, 1973): 1, 3.

40. Rosemary Stevens, *American Medicine and the Public Interest* (New Haven: Yale University Press, 1971), pp. 362-67; Florence A. Wilson and Duncan Neuhauser, *Health Services in the United States* (Cambridge: Ballinger, 1974), pp. 118-19, 163-65.

41. Data culled from U.S. Department of Health, Education, and Welfare, Public Health Service, Health Resources Administration, *Health Professions Schools: Selected B.H.M. Support Data F.Y. 1965-1967* (Washington, D.C.: Department of Health, Education, and Welfare, 1977), p. 120.

42. Institute of Medicine, *Costs of Education in the Health Professions* (Bethesda, Md.: National Academy of Sciences, U.S. Department of Health, Education, and Welfare, Public Health Service, Health Resources Administration, Bureau of Health Resources Development, 1974), pp. xiv, xviii.

43. Data culled from catalogs of the colleges for the respective years.

44. For latest published information on characteristics of osteopathic faculty, see American Association of Colleges of Osteopathic Medicine, *Final Report of the Osteopathic Medical Manpower Information Project,* pp. 47-54.

45. "Michigan Plans New College," *AOA News Bull.* 6 (May 1963): 1; "Michigan College Site Moved from Lansing to Pontiac," *AOA News Bull.* 7 (December 1964): 1.

46. "Michigan College Moves Two Steps," *AOA News Bull.* 8 (August 1965): 3; "Michigan Study Cites Role of D.O.'s," *AOA News Bull.* 4 (August 1961): 3; "Plan for Health Care Drafted in Michigan," *AOA News Bull.* 5 (September 1962): 4.

47. "Michigan College Moves Two Steps," p. 3.

48. "Michigan D.O.'s Vote 87 Percent against Merger," *AOA News Bull.* 9 (April 1969): 1-2.

49. "Michigan to Establish Osteopathic School," *AOA News Review* 12 (August 1969): 1-2.

50. Ibid., p. 2; see also John Walsh, "Medicine at Michigan State," *Science* 177 (1972): 1085-87; *Science* 178 (1972): 36-39, 288-91, 377-80.

51. "T.C.O.M. Becomes State-Supported Medical School as Governor Briscoe Signs S.B. 216," *Texas Osteopathic Physicians Journal* 32 (July 1975): 12-13; "Basic Science Education Agreement Signed with State University," *The D.O.* 12 (April 1972): 171; "T.C.O.M. Receives Government Funding in Excess of $800,000," *The D.O.* 13 (October 1972): 201-2; "State Grants $3.4 Million Appropriation for T.C.O.M.," *The D.O.* 13 (August 1973): 202.

52. "Preliminary Study Shows Feasibility of Osteopathic College in Oklahoma," *The D.O.* 12 (December 1971): 114-15; "New Osteopathic College Slated for Oklahoma," *The D.O.* 12 (April, 1972): 99; "Legislature Appropriates Funds for Oklahoma Osteopathic College," *The D.O.* 12 (May 1972): 90-91.

53. Carol R. Thiessen, "Greenbriar: The Little College that Could," *The D.O.* 15 (March 1975): 86-92; "West Virginia Now a State College," *The D.O.* 15 (May 1975): 130.

54. Carol R. Thiessen, "And Now There Are Ten," *The D.O.* 17 (September 1976): 85.

55. Jeff Kressman, "New Colleges Open in New Jersey, New York," *The D.O.* 18 (March 1978): 33-37.

56. Edward P. Crowell, "Accelerating Educational Growth Dominates Board Session," *The D.O.* 18 (April 1978): 46.

57. Carol R. Thiessen, "California Supreme Court Reopens the Golden State to Licensure," *The D.O.* 18 (April 1978): 46.

58. U.S. Department of Health, Education, and Welfare, Public Health Service, Health Resources Administration, Office of Graduate Medical Education, *Interim Report of the Graduate Medical Education National Advisory Committee to the Secretary* (Hyattsville, Md.: Department of Health, Education, and Welfare, 1979), p. 161.

## Chapter 10: The Present and the Future

1. Edward P. Crowell, "Report of the Executive Director," *The D.O.* 16 (November 1975): 75; Donald Siehl, "A.O.A. President's Address," *The D.O.* 19 (August 1979): 19-21.

2. Leonard D. Fenninger and Rose H. Tracy, "Graduate Medical Education," in *Medical Education in the United States, 1973-74*, ed. Anne E. Crowley (Chicago: American Medical Association, 1975), p. 35.

3. "Hospital Requirements for Intern Training and the Intern Registration Program," *JAOA* 76 (April 1977) supplement: 119-25.

4. Norman Gevitz, "Osteopathic Internship and Residency Programs: A Statistical Report" (Paper presented to the Liaison Committee on Osteopathic Information, American Association of Colleges of Osteopathic Medicine, Washington, D.C., 1975).

5. Edward P. Crowell, "A.O.A. Board and House Approve Special Assessment," *The D.O.* 18 (October 1975): 55-61; idem, "Board, House Respond to Small States' Concerns," *The D.O.* 18 (October 1977): 37-39.

6. Incomplete data for 1979-80 would indicate that there are 10 percent more positions

than nonmilitary-bound graduates to fill them. See the "Fact Sheet," in *The D.O.* 20 (November 1979): 119-20.

7. Recent data indicate that the number of D.O.'s in AMA-approved training programs is up sharply. In 1977 there were 386, in 1980, 741. This near-doubling clearly reflects the dramatic expansion in the number of osteopathic graduates. It would appear, though, that the great majority of these D.O.'s are in such programs with AOA approval. Of the latter figure, 237 are in federal internships and residencies. See American Medical Association, *'81/'82 Directory of Residency Training Programs* (Chicago: AMA, 1981), p. 60.

8. "Policy Statement of the A.O.A. Board on Certificates of Need," *The D.O.* 15 (April 1975): 59-61; Edward P. Crowell, "Report of the Executive Director," *The D.O.* 16 (November 1975): 75-76; "Maine Legislation Favors D.O.'s," *The D.O.* 18 (August 1978): 61.

9. Edward P. Crowell, "Osteopathic Education Dominates Cincinnati Meeting," *The D.O.* 19 (October 1978): 62-64; John C. Taylor, "Washington Report," *The D.O.* 17 (April 1977): 37; "A.O.A. Newsbriefs," *The D.O.* 20 (December 1979): 11.

10. Jack Leahy, "Manipulation: A Survey of How D.O.'s Feel about It," *O.P.* 38 (March 1972): 31-36. National Center for Health Statistics, *Office Visits to Osteopathic Physicians, Jan.-Dec. 1974: Provisional Data from the National Ambulatory Medical Care Survey* (Washington, n.d.), p. 19.

11. Spencer G. Bradford, "The Application of Osteopathic Manipulative Therapy," in *Osteopathic Medicine,* ed. J. Marshall Hoag, Wilbur V. Cole and Spencer G. Bradford (New York: McGraw Hill, 1969), p. 179.

12. American Osteopathic Association, "Guide to the Function of the Committee on the Utilization of Osteopathic Principles and Practices," mimeographed (Chicago, 1972), p. 1.

13. Edward G. Stiles, "Osteopathic Manipulation in a Hospital Environment," *JAOA* 76 (1976): 243-58; Mary J. Cramblit, "A.O.A. Convention Considers Osteopathic Hospital Distinctiveness," *The D.O.* 18 (February 1978): 53-56; Waterville Osteopathic Hospital, "Informational Package on the Osteopathic Manipulative Medical Service" (Waterville, Maine, n.d.).

14. Ira C. Rumney, "Specialization in Osteopathic Manipulative Medicine," *Osteopathic Annals* 4 (April 1975): 12-17. Also in the same issue of the *Annals:* Norman J. Larson, "Certification in Osteopathic Manipulative Medicine," pp. 28-29; J. P. Wood, "Is Certification the Answer?" pp. 30-35; Elliot L. Hix, "Another View on Specialty Recognition for Osteopathic Manipulative Medicine," pp. 36-39; Philip E. Greenman, "Competency in Palpating Diagnosis and Treatment," pp. 18-27.

15. See Murray Goldstein, ed., *The Research Status of Spinal Manipulative Therapy* (Bethesda, Md.: Department of Health, Education, and Welfare, Public Health Service, National Institutes of Health, National Institute of Neurological and Communicative Disorders and Stroke, 1975), and Irwin M. Korr, ed., *The Neurobiologic Mechanisms in Manipulative Therapy* (New York: Plenum Press, 1978).

16. See Myron S. Magen, "The Osteopathic Short Leg Syndrome: Research," *The D.O.* 17 (June 1977): 93-97; J. Jerry Rodos, "The Second Century of Osteopathic Research," *The D.O.* 19 (June 1979): 43-49.

17. "The D.O. Needs an Image," *O.P.* 36 (April 1969): 14-22. Because of the manner in which these results were reported it can only be assumed that the remaining respondents to this last question answered either "the same" or "unsure."

18. Stephen Shortell, "Occupational Prestige Differences within the Medical and Allied Health Professions," *Social Science and Medicine* 8 (1974): 1-9.

19. Personal communication from Professor Shortell to me.

20. Burson-Marsteller Research," A Survey of Public Attitudes towards Medical Care and Medical Professionals Prepared for the American Osteopathic Association," typescript (March 1981).

21. Jack Leahy, "How D.O.'s Feel about Their 'Image,'" *O.P.* 40 (September 1973): 37-

43; Jack Leahy, "Should Our Schools Alter Their D.O. Degree Policy?" *O.P.* 37 (April 1971): 9-21; *O.P.* 38 (January 1972): 47-53.

22. Jack Leahy, "Georgia D.O. Wins Suit to Use M.D. Suffix," *O.P.* 40 (August 1973): 31; "Georgia D.O. R. T. Oliver Has Right to Use M.D. If Georgia Composite Board Wants to Grant Licenses to F.M.G.'s with Same Designation," *AMA News* 16 (July 30, 1973): 3, 7.

23. "Editorial Comment: Dismissal of Oliver Suit in New York and New Jersey," *JAOA* 78 (1978): 97; Thaddeus P. Kawalak, "A New Look at the D.O. Degree," *O.P.* 46 (March 1979): 41-44.

24. "Editorial: The A.M.A.'s 'Report D,'" *JAOA* 74 (1975): 602-3; "Plan to License D.O.'s is Rejected," *American Medical News* 17 (December 9, 1974): 20.

25. "California Bill Would Permit D.O.'s to Become M.D.'s," *American Medical News* 21 (August 4, 1978): 11; Kawalak, "New Look at the D.O. Degree," p. 44; "Dismissal of Oliver Suit in New York and New Jersey," p. 176; "Objective: Destruction," *JAOA* 77 (1978): 895; "A Matter of Degrees," *JAOA* 78 (1978): 547-49. "Plan Delayed to License D.O.'s as M.D.'s," *American Medical News* 23 (March 4, 1980): 1, 3.

26. In a three-hour NBC special aired January 3, 1978, entitled *Medicine in America,* the D.O.'s were not mentioned until the closing minutes of the program, when they were lumped together with the chiropractors as subjects which the narrator said they unfortunately did not have time to cover. This neglect drew an unprecedented number of angry letters and phone calls to the AOA Public Relations Office, which had tried without success while the show was being prepared to have the profession included. See Edward P. Crowell, "Accelerating Educational Growth Dominates Board Session," *The D.O.* 18 (April 1978): 52-53.

27. George W. Northup, "Editorial: 'Down the Tube—to Where?'" *JAOA* 78 (1978): 251.

# *Index*

Academy of Applied Osteopathy, 94
Ackerknecht, E., 6
Adjuncts, 64-66
Advertising, 36-37
Allopathy, 8
American Association of Medical Colleges, 101-2, 115
American College of Surgeons, 81
American Hospital Association, 122-23
American Medical Association: inspection of osteopathic schools by, 103-10; policy of, toward osteopathy, 110, 112, 117-20, 123-29
American Osteopathic Association: and AMA inspection of osteopathic schools, 103-10; and California Osteopathic Association, 112-16; code of ethics of, 55-57; combating impostors and imitators, 57-60; on the D.O. degree, 97-98; early legislative efforts of, 49-50; establishing the *Journal,* 53; formation of, 48; lengthening the course of study, 50-52; membership of, 57; on osteopathic principles in hospitals, 89; resisting the AMA, 117-20, 124-29; sponsoring research, 54-55; on teaching of *materia medica,* 70-74; and teaching of osteopathy, 142-43; on unaccredited degrees, 102
American School of Osteopathy; early classes of, 28; early relations of, with other schools, 45-47; expanded curriculum of, 28; expansion of facilities in, 80; Flexner on, 78; formation of, 19; initial training provided in, 19-23; introduction of surgery and obstetrics in, 61-64; opposing the three-year course, 52;

teaching of vaccine and serum therapy in, 70. *See also* Kirksville College of Osteopathic Medicine
Appel, James Z., 108
Apprenticeship system, 4
Ashmore, Edythe, 53
Associated Colleges of Osteopathy, 50-51
Atlantic School of Osteopathy, 44, 52

Babbitt, Edwin Dwight, 13
Bacot, John, 30
Bailly, Jean Sylvan, 12
Balfour, William, 30
Bane Report, 130
*Banner of Light,* 13
Barber, Elmer, 45-46
Barber, Helen, 45-46
Basic science boards, 82, 86-87
Bayne-Jones Report, 130
Beach, Wooster, 9
Bernard, Herbert, 36, 65
Bigelow, Jacob, 6
Blauch, L. E., 83
Bloodletting, 5
Bonesetting, 15-16
Booth, Eamons R., 51-52
Botanical medicine, 7-9
Bradford, Spencer G., 141
Braid, James, 12
"Broad osteopaths," 61
Bronk, Detlev, 91
Brown, Pat, 115
Brown, Thomas, 32
Brown-Sequard, C. E., 32-33
Bunting, Henry Stanhope, 56, 70-71, 90

179

Burns, Louisa, 54-55, 90-91
Bushnell, Horace, 1

California College of Medicine. *See* College of Osteopathic Physicians and Surgeons
California College of Osteopathy, 52
California Medical Association, 101, 112, 114-16, 120-21, 147
California merger, 99-102, 112-16; aftermath of, 117-22
California Osteopathic Association, 101-3, 111-16
Calomel, 5-6
Case reports, 53-54
Central College of Osteopathy, 78
Chandler, Louis, 93
Chandler, L. R., 108
Chicago College of Osteopathy, 51, 62, 69-70, 73, 78, 80, 84, 103, 130, 131-32
Chiropractic, 58-60, 86-87
Christian Science, 13
Cleobury, W., 30
Cline, John W., 104, 105, 106, 107
Cluett, Therese, 36, 38
College of Osteopathic Medicine and Surgery. *See* Des Moines Still College of Osteopathy and Surgery
College of Osteopathic Medicine of the Pacific, 135-36
College of Osteopathic Physicians and Surgeons, 52, 62, 70, 80, 81, 84, 85, 99, 100, 115, 121, 124
Collins, Harry L., 62-63
Colorado College of Osteopathy, 52
Columbian School of Osteopathy, 46-47
Comprehensive Health Manpower Training Act of 1971, 130
Comstock, E. S., 73

Davis, Andrew Jackson, 13
Deason, John, 54
DeLenderecie, Helen, 42
Denslow, J. Stedman, 90-92
D.O. degree, 97-98, 145-48
Des Moines Still College of Osteopathy and Surgery, 44, 45, 78, 80, 84, 125, 130, 132

Drugs: displacing distinctive osteopathic procedures, 93-94; introduction of study of, in curriculum, 66-74

Eccles, A. J., 30
Eclecticism, 9
Eddy, Mary Baker, 13
Education: and the addition of pharmacology into the curriculum, 66-74; and comparison of M.D. and D.O. schools, 75-80; decline in distinctive osteopathic elements of, 88-94; and development of new schools, 132-36; and establishment of early colleges, 43-47; federal aid to, 130; financial basis of, 79-80; and improved financial status of colleges, 130-32; improving standards of, 82-85; and internships and residencies, 85-86; and introduction of surgery and obstetrics in curriculum, 61-64; lengthening the course of study, 50-52; and problems of college expansion, 137-41
Etherington, Frederick, 83
Evans, A. L., 37-38, 39
Evans, Warren Felt, 13

Fake degrees, 98
Federal service of D.O.'s, 124, 126
Federation of State Medical Boards, 101
Fishbein, Morris, 102
Flexner, Abraham, 76-78
Foley, L. Alice, 96
Foraker, Senator, 25
Foreign medical graduates, 86-87
Franklin, Benjamin, 12
French Academy of Medicine, 12
French Academy of Sciences, 12
Furry, Frank J., 68-69

Gaddis, Cyrus, 96
Gerard, Ralph Waldo, 91
Graham, Douglas, 30, 31
Graham, Sylvester, 10-11
Greenwood, P. F., 26
Gregg, Alan, 90
Grunigan, Forest, 101

Hahnemann, Samuel, 8
Hammond, William, 6
Hannah, F. W., 38
Harris, Wilfred, 51
Hartman, George, 95
Hazzard, Charles, 29, 31-32, 33
Health Manpower Act of 1968, 130
Health Professions Educational Act of 1963, 130
Heatherington, J. Scott, 127
Helmer, George, 41-42
Henderson, Elmer, 103
Heroic therapy, 5-7, 11
Hildreth, Arthur, 50
Hill-Burton Act, 85
Hilton, John, 32
Hinckle, W. A., 68
Holistic medicine, 142
Holmes, Oliver Wendell, Sr., 6, 9
Hood, Wharton, 16
Homeopathy, 7-8
Hospitals, 78, 80, 81, 84-86, 89, 121, 138, 141
Hulett, C.M.T., 51, 65
Hulett, M. F., 96
Hydropathy, 11
Hypnosis, 12

Impostors, 57-58
Influenza pandemic of 1918-19, 71-72

Jenner, Edward, 7
Joint Commission on the Accreditation of Hospitals, 123
*Journal of Osteopathy,* 23-24
*Journal of the American Osteopathic Association,* 53

Kansas City College of Osteopathy and Surgery, 80, 84, 85, 130, 132
Keesecker, Raymond, 97
Kinsman, J. Murray, 108
Kirksville, 14, 23-25
Kirksville College of Osteopathic Medicine, 84, 85, 130, 132. *See also* American School of Osteopathy
Kisch, Arnold I., 114

Koch, Robert, 33
Korr, Irwin M., 91-92, 144

Lane, James, 3
Larson, Leonard, 108
Laughlin, George, 79
Lavoisier, Antoine, 12
Legan, Marshall Scott, 11
Legislation: and achievement of full licensure, 137; early struggles with, 39-42; and the effect of improving educational standards, 81-87; the independent board movement, 49-50; and *materia medica,* 73; in Missouri, 26-29
"Lesion osteopaths," 61
Licensure. *See* Legislation
Ling, Peter Henry, 31
Littlejohn, David, 29
Littlejohn, James, 29, 64
Littlejohn, J. Martin, 29, 32, 51
Los Angeles College of Osteopathy, 52, 69, 78, 99
Los Angeles County Osteopathic Hospital, 100

McConnell, Carl P., 29, 33, 66
McCormack, John, 40
McNamara, Robert, 124
Magnetic healing, 12-15
Marsh, Dorothy, 114
Massachusetts College of Osteopathy, 51, 69, 70, 78
Massage, 29-31
*Materia medica. See* Drugs
Matthews, S. C., 57
Medicare, 124
*Merck Manual of Therapeutics,* 67
Mesmer, Franz, 12
Methodist church, 1-2, 10
"Metropolitan University," 102
Michigan Association of Osteopathic Physicians and Surgeons, 133
"Michigan Resolution," 113
Michigan State Medical Society, 137
Michigan State University College of Osteopathic Medicine, 132-34
Milwaukee College of Osteopathy, 52
"Mind Cure," 13

lumbian School of Osteopathy, 47; in
defense of the term osteopathy, 35; establishment of infirmary by, 18; on germ
theory, 33; as "lightning bonesetter," 15-
18; as magnetic healer, 12-15; medical
education and practice of, 4-7; opening
of school by, 19; opposing *materia med-
ica,* 71; teaching of, 19-23; on vaccines
and serums, 66-67; view of drugless
methods, 10-11; view of homeopathy
and eclecticism, 9-10, 23
Still, Charles, 40, 52, 67
Still, George A., 63-64
Still, Harry, 17-18
Still, Martha, 1
Stone, Governor, 28
Sullivan, Joseph, 38
Sullivan, Mark, 97
Surgery, 61-64
Swedish Movements, 31-32
Sweet, William, 2
Sweet family, 16
Swieten, Gerald von, 30
"Sympathies," 32

Tasker, Dain, 64-65
Taylor, George H., 30-31

Taylor, S. L., 64
Teall, Charles C., 69
Texas College of Osteopathic Medicine,
134-35
Thomson, Samuel, 7-8

United States Civil Service Commission,
124

Vaccines, 67
Viseltear, Arthur, 114

Ward, Marcus, 46-47
Washington state merger attempt, 120
Waterville Osteopathic Hospital, 143
Wescoe, W. Clarke, 108
West Virginia School of Osteopathic Med-
icine, 135
Whiting, Lillian, 62
Women students, 44-45
Woodbury, G. W., 89

Young, C. W., 65
Young, Frank P., 64

*The Johns Hopkins University Press*

THE D.O.'s

This book was composed in Times Roman text and display type by David Lorton from a design by Lisa S. Mirski. It was printed on S. D. Warren's 50-lb. Sebago Eggshell paper and bound in Kivar 5 by Universal Lithographers, Inc.